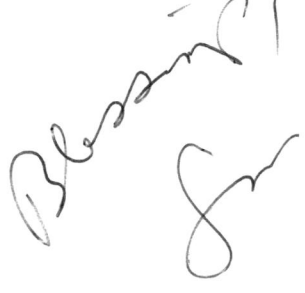

MW01613281

The Victory Is Pure Joy

"I have fought the good fight. I have finished the race.
I have kept the faith."
— 2 Timothy 4:7

Sandy Rice

Fairway Press, Lima, Ohio

THE VICTORY IS PURE JOY

FIRST EDITION
Copyright © 2001 by
Sandy Rice

All rights reserved. No portion of this book may be reproduced or utilized in any form or by any means, electronic or mechanical including photocopying, without permission in writing from the publisher. Inquiries should be addressed to: Fairway Press, 517 South Main Street, P.O. Box 4503, Lima, Ohio 45802-4503.

All scripture quotations are taken from the Holy Bible, New International Version. Copyright (c) 1973, 1978, 1984 International Bible Society. Used by permission of Zondervan Bible Publishers. All rights reserved.

ISBN 0-7880-2006-4   PRINTED IN U.S.A.

This book is dedicated to our darling granddaughter, Amanda Brooke Rice. She has brought into our lives the greatest of joys. God gave her to our family in His perfect timing, when we all needed great healing for our broken hearts. She will always be a reminder of God's faithfulness to our family and of His never failing love for us.

In Appreciation

I want to thank my husband, Jim, our sons, Andrew and Adam and their precious wives, Julie and Rita, for their unfailing support and encouragement. God has blessed us with the most wonderful family in the world and I will never cease to praise Him for each of them. I first thank them for their love for the Lord and then for their love for one another and for me. I love each of you deeply!

I want to especially thank Louise Nielsen for so much. Where do I begin? She has been my editor, my sounding board, my critic and most of all my friend! I could not have completed this book without her help. She has expended much time, money and energy to get it to the publisher. Lou, I love you and I am sincerely indebted to you for your love and support.

A heartfelt thank-you to Debby Weidman and Sherry Neuenschwander for all the help and support you were to me and to my family over these past difficult years. For the tireless assistance you provided in the marketing of my first book and for all the help you were in the care of Joy. You are blessings and I love you both.

I thank Zelda Artz for her constant encouragement to me and to our family over these past four years. Her love for us and her vigilant prayers have sustained and kept us. I love you very much, Zel.

To our church family at Faith Presbyterian Church of Kingstowne, Virginia, I thank you and praise God for you.

To Teri, Kevin and Tyler, I thank you for making Joy's last days in your home so wonderful. She loved you all so much! We blended our families together to care for and nurture Joy through the most difficult challenge of her life and I know she was happy and grateful for that. May God richly bless you!

To Renee Brooks of Fairway Press and to all those at CSS, I thank you for caring enough to see that my books were published and so beautifully finished. I appreciate being given the opportunity to share this story of hope and encouragement to others.

***

In Memory

In memory of my sister-in-law, Joanne Rushworth Bostetter who fought her battle with breast cancer for six years until the Lord called her home, June 12, 2001. Joanne and Joy had been a comfort and support to one another and now they are together with our Lord and Savior, Jesus Christ.

Foreword

Sandy Rice hopes that the sharing of her experiences will afford a glimpse into the inner workings of a family sold out to God ... that her writing will examine, as under a microscope, the spiritual growth incurred by pain ... and that *The Victory Is Pure Joy* will touch readers with hope to press on through their own trials of faith.

As Sandy traces Joy's path from independence to dependence, she accomplishes all of those objectives and more. As a counselor, I commend her for spotlighting the need for emotional support from "the household of faith."

"What a wonderful God we have — He is the Father of our Lord Jesus Christ, the source of every mercy, and the One who so wonderfully comforts and strengthens us in our hardships and trials. And why does He do this? So that when others are troubled, needing our sympathy and encouragement, we can pass on to them this same help and comfort God has given us" (2 Corinthians 1:3-5, The Living Bible).

The truth of one of my favorite quotes comes to life in these chapters: "Joy is not the absence of pain, but the presence of God." I will suggest this book to those struggling with grief and loss issues as an aid in finding God's healing.

Joy Jacobs
Author and Counselor
Shepherd's Touch Counseling Ministries

The Victory Is Pure Joy

To have known Joy Seale, even for a short time, was pure joy. I arrived on the scene rather late, but will always be grateful for the privilege of knowing Joy and being her pastor at Faith Evangelical Presbyterian Church in the last two years of her earthly life. An inspiration to all who knew her and her courageous fight against cancer, Joy gave us a living example of what it means to walk by faith, not by sight. For she was fully persuaded that even in the valley of death's dark shadow, God was with her, just as He promised in His Word (Psalm 23:4). Even while losing her battle with cancer, Joy proved to be more than a conqueror through the Lord Jesus Christ, who loved her and gave Himself for her (Romans 8:37).

To know Sandy Rice with her vibrant faith in Christ, her quick sense of humor, her indomitable spirit, and her loving heart, is pure joy as well. If joy, as C.S. Lewis observed, is the serious business of heaven, then Sandy Rice is one serious Christian, for it is evident to all who know her that the joy of the Lord is her strength (Nehemiah 8:10). I count myself blessed to be her pastor.

I praise God for the testimonies of these two women and their unwavering faith. May you be blessed and encouraged by their story. This book is a gift to be cherished, for in it, even though she is dead, Joy still speaks. Thanks be to God, who gives us the victory, through Jesus Christ our Lord (1 Corinthians 15:57).

Pastor Neil Smith
Faith Evangelical Presbyterian Church

***

I feel honored to have had the opportunity to have known Joy, and to have been blessed by her witness to God's amazing grace through her eight long years of struggle with the ravages of one of earth's enemies, cancer.

Sandy has captured the true meaning for our earthly walk as she ministered to Joy as friend, spiritual mentor, caretaker, and sister in the Lord. Sandy showed her deep devotion to her Lord and Savior, Jesus Christ, as she shared her faith, life, family, home, and loving care for Joy, as well as her aging mother, until they each entered into the presence of their Lord. I have had the personal privilege of experiencing the deep friendship and love of Sandy, her husband Jim, and their family and I hope you are blessed as well, as you enjoy reading of the victory through much sacrifice and love for others.

Joy fought the good fight, kept the faith, and blessed so many others by her witness to God's amazing grace. Sandy was a shining example for us, as she followed the teaching of the Apostle Paul when he wrote to the Philippians: "If you have any encouragement from being united with Christ, if any comfort from his love, if any fellowship with the Spirit, if any tenderness and compassion, then make my joy complete by being like-minded, having the same love, being one in spirit and purpose. Do nothing out of selfish ambition or vain conceit, but in humility consider others better than yourself" (Philippians 2:1-3).

Your faith will be strengthened and your joy will be complete, as you witness God's wonderful all sufficient grace.

Zelda Artz, Elder and Sister in Christ
Faith Evangelical Presbyterian Church
Kingstowne, Virginia

***

John 15:12-14 reads, "Love each other as I have loved you. Greater love has no one than this, that he lay down his life for his friends. You are my friends if you do what I command."

This passage in John paints a beautiful picture of true friendship. It's this kind of sacrificial friendship that I have seen between my sister, Sandy, and Joy. Sandy was always there for Joy even before the diagnosis of cancer was made. After the diagnosis Sandy devoted herself to being not only Joy's friend, but her caregiver, as well.

As a nurse, I know the great responsibility of the caregiver's role for a cancer patient and how difficult it is. When the patient is your best friend, the role must seem impossible. But not with Sandy. She walked beside Joy every step of the way. She was her friend, teacher, cheerleader, nurse, counselor, prayer partner, and sister in Christ. She went with Joy to doctor appointments and chemotherapy, helped her make decisions, gave her injections, helped her with her medication, made special food for her, laughed and cried with her, and sat by her bedside giving comfort and reassurance of God's love when pain and fear set in.

Before Joy's death Sandy helped Joy plan her "celebration of life" service and spoke at length with her about Heaven and what would be waiting for her there.

I love my sister, Sandy, and I am proud of her for giving herself so unselfishly to the needs of her friend. Her books were written for one purpose only ... to teach us how we can be an extension of God's loving hands for others and how we can follow His commandment.

Sandy, big sister, you have taught me a lot throughout life. Thank you for teaching me this very valuable lesson — "Greater love hath no one than this, that he lay down his life for his friends."

Your Loving Sister,
Carolyn

***

After hearing the news of my friend's recent diagnosis with breast cancer, I realized the understandable amount of sadness, she must have been feeling. I wanted to give her encouragement, by making a cancer survivor video. Several cancer survivors from Internet Support groups and from the American Cancer Society contacted me. One survivor in particular offered encouragement and suggested a book that would be beneficial to me in caring for

Sue. Immediately, I visited the local Barnes and Noble bookstore, in hopes of finding this book. To my dismay, they did not carry this book. I skimmed through several of the offered titles. None appealed to me. Turning to leave the aisle, I glanced down at the bottom shelf and was drawn to a book called To Run The Race With Joy. *I purchased it. While reading the book, I experienced an array of emotions, as Joy's story was told. The spiritual aspects that were displayed in this book were invaluable. Desiring to learn more, I decided to contact the writer, Sandy Rice. Sandy and I spoke for quite some time and I was inspired by her Godly perspective.*

I know God put Sandy and her book in our lives for a purpose. I know these events were not by coincidence, rather, I truly believe they were all planned and directed by God. Sandy's book inspired me to continue on in my endeavor. I am grateful to Sandy for writing with such care, and to Joy, for modeling such faithfulness. I have been greatly anticipating The Victory Is Pure Joy *to continue the story of a wonderful and courageous woman I have grown to admire.*

Christina Morales
Gainsville, VA

* * *

I met Joy many years ago in our church youth group. She was a few years older than I but I knew as soon as I met her that I was going to like her. She was funny, loud, a great athlete but also kind and sensitive. She was a new Christian and really wanted to have Christ as the centerpiece of her life. We were both taught many things by our youth leader, Sandy Rice, and her husband, Jim. They ministered to us in such a unique way as I look back on it now. Sandy was a "very real" Christian. She actually lived her faith and love for Christ each and every day and in each and every area of her life. That was something that Joy and I really looked up to.

As we got older and moved on through high school and college, I saw Joy's relationship with Sandy and her family turn into a deeply devoted friendship. Joy needed stability in her life and the

Rices met her need. When Joy developed breast cancer, they became her support system especially after her parents died. Joy kept her laughter and smile whenever I saw her as did Sandy's family. God kept them all strong for one another. Wow! What a powerful network God put together.

Lori Jeffries Murnane,
Immanuel Bible Church, Springfield, VA

***

As you were there for Joy, Sandy, I thank you for being there for me during the darkest hours of my life. Your love, caring and support gave me the strength to get through that most difficult time. Your friendship has been a blessing and a gift from God and one that I'll always cherish. Your books are a wonderful inspiration to everyone who reads them.

Love,
Mary Montano
Groveton Baptist Church, Alexandria, VA

Introduction

When Joy Seale was fourteen years of age, I led her to a saving faith in Jesus Christ as her personal Lord and Savior. Through her adolescence, I counseled and discipled her as she grew in the knowledge of the Lord. Little did I know that our lives would be knit together forever when she was diagnosed with breast cancer at the young age of 35.

Joy's parents died in 1993 and our family became her family as we became her primary caregivers. I wrote my first book, *To Run The Race With Joy*, published in 1997, chronicling our struggles with Joy's cancer and her marvelous testimony in the face of that struggle, from the time she was diagnosed in 1991, until 1995, when all seemed fairly settled.

Sadly, the "remission" proved to be short-lived and Joy's cancer returned with fury. *The Victory Is Pure Joy* completes this glorious testimony to God's amazing grace and to his all-sufficient strength in the face of one crisis after another, while also giving to us one blessing after another.

And so with tears of joy mingling with tears of pain, I complete for you the remarkable story of our race with Joy and her final victory....

***

Joyful Reflections: Joy was excited about my idea to incorporate her thoughts into *The Victory Is Pure Joy*. She was able to complete her first 20 "Joyful Reflections" before she died. The remainder were taken directly from her journal and notes written in her daily devotions. Joy kept her journal up-to-date until February 14, 1999.

Chapter 1

His Continual Amazing Grace

Oh, that I could tell you that Joy has been healed of her cancer! What I would give to be able to relay to you all the miraculous healing that God has accomplished in her body! But, I cannot do that. It has not been God's will for her life. What I can share with you is a continuation of God's marvelous grace to each of us as we ran the race with Joy.

Let me take you back to the summer of 1995. Our family vacation came and went, and as usual it was filled with wonderful memories that I will cherish for a long time to come. I praise the Lord that even with all of our sorrows over these past few years, our summers at the beach have been precious and Joy has felt unusually well during those blessed times. We have all needed the relaxation, and the fact that she felt good had a therapeutic effect on us all.

I continued to give her the painful injections three times weekly to help keep her blood count up. They continued to be just as painful for me as they had always been. I prayed for an easier way!

I felt as though we were suspended in space. The stem cell transplant that she had gone through in December of 1993, had not been successful! The cancer was ever present and hovering over her body, but not moving one way or the other. I thanked the Lord daily that at least it was not spreading. There was still the cancer-related fluid on her left lung and her cough persisted. I prayed that the cancer didn't invade her lungs! She still took weekly chemotherapy, the 5FU with vitamins, and it appeared to be keeping the cancer in check. Again, I had to thank God for the chemotherapy

15

even though I knew it destroyed and weakened her body (just as surely as did the cancer), still, it was keeping her alive!

I kept reminding myself daily of God's word and I knew that although cancer may destroy her body, it could not destroy her spirit! He is our portion in times of discouragement.

Psalm 16:11 promises, *"You have made known to me the path of life; you will fill me with joy in your presence...."*

Joyful Reflections - 1

I had always prayed that God would allow me the privilege of living until *To Run The Race With Joy* was published. Praise Him for His amazing grace because He did grant my desire to witness that and to be part of a ministry that I have loved so much. He evidently has more that He wants me to do for Him before He calls me home.

Each morning when I open my eyes, I thank God for yet another day of mercy and opportunities for service for Him, and for His amazing grace that permits me to experience that new day and the blessings and challenges it will bring. My spirit is at rest in God alone even though the cancer still races through my body.

I now can thank Him for my cancer because through it I have been drawn so much closer to Him. Cancer cannot destroy my spirit or my soul!

Chapter 2

Go Redskins, Go!

In late August of 1995, Joy called me at work one day with excitement bubbling in her voice. "What are you doing on September 3 around 4:00 in the afternoon?"

"Well," I said in a bewildered voice, "I don't really know. What did you have in mind?"

"Guess what I have in my hot little hands right now?" she playfully asked.

"I don't know. What do you have in your hot little hands right now? I give up. Tell me, nimnut," I replied, using our word for "nitwit," "numskull" and "nut" all rolled into one!

"I have," she gleefully continued while stretching the news out as long as she possibly could, "two tickets. That is two, as in not one but two, tickets to ..." She abruptly stopped. "Oh, don't you want to guess at least one guess?"

"No! I do not have time for games," I stated, becoming just a little annoyed because she had caught me in the middle of getting my office set up for the beginning of the school year!

"Well," she continued, undaunted by my attempt at being annoyed, "I have tickets to the opening game of the Redskins 1996 season! Now what do you think of that? I thought we could have ladies day out and you and I could go. Good idea?"

I was ecstatic about the prospects of going to a real game. We had been to a pre-season game, but never to a real game. "Are you kidding?" I yelled. "Of course we will go! Adam will be back in school then and Jim, Mom, Julie and Andrew can watch us on TV! Do you think we can get close enough to a camera to take a sign that says, 'Happy Birthday, Adam'? After all, September 3 will be his 21st birthday! Wouldn't that be great if while he is watching the game in the dorm, he would see our sign?"

I could just picture us there at the game with our sign held high and everyone knowing that it was my son's birthday. I could feel the adrenaline pulsing through my veins. What a day we would have.

We chattered and plotted for a while and really psyched ourselves up. So much so that it was hard to get back to my completely cluttered clinic that had to be in top shape before I could go home. I hummed the Redskins' fight song and before too long I had the job completed and my office was ready for the 1995-96 school year and the hundreds of students that would be coming through my doors in a few short days.

I pray for those students to whom God allows me to minister each day. I treat each one of them, regardless of their background or color, as if they were my own. There are such deep needs in our young people today. If they only realized that Christ is the answer. I try to show them all the love and care that I can, and over the years I have been able to witness to many of them of God's deep concern and love for them. I have tried to plant many seeds and I know that God has honored that. The students know my standards and what my life is all about and my moral code of conduct. And even though some of them think I am very old-fashioned, I know that they respect me for my honesty. I only wish I could do more to help them.

The day of the game arrived and Jim, Julie and Andrew drove us to the metrorail station where we boarded the metro dressed up in our best Redskins clothing. We carried a huge posterboard sign with our birthday greeting printed in large letters, "HAPPY 21st BIRTHDAY, ADAM, LONGWOOD COLLEGE."

"Getting that into the metro car will be very interesting," Joy said sarcastically. "But it is your responsibility to carry it without ripping it apart."

"Okay. I'll do it. I'll just keep it rolled up," I stated with staunch authority in my voice!

Once we got to the stadium, excitement filled the air as all of the fans pressed towards the gate. We got caught up in the crowd and were soon talking to complete strangers about the game. We were all there with one common purpose — to cheer our team on to victory in this, the opening game of the season! It makes me wonder what would happen if Christians would all band together with one purpose — to proclaim Jesus Christ with this same kind of enthusiasm! My, what a changed world we would have!

Our seats were great except that they were up pretty high into the stands — the nosebleed section. Joy grew very tired as we climbed and climbed and climbed until we reached our destination. However, the smile on her face because of the anticipation of what was to come belied the pain that I knew she was feeling with every step she took.

We settled down and watched our team, as well as the opposing team, the Arizona Cardinals, warm up and we cheered as loudly as we possibly could as the Redskins left the field for the locker room. The stadium fairly rocked a short while later, as we stood for the team introductions and the National Anthem.

"We" were in control of the game from the beginning, much to the delight of Joy and me as well as all of our new "friends" around us. We did the "wave," high-fived each other and generally yelled our lungs out with every great play and touchdown. It was great! I looked over at her radiant face several times and thanked God for allowing us to make yet another memory that even time can't erase.

At half-time we decided to find the NBC local cameraman and ask if we could get our sign on television. We made our way over to the other side of the stadium and when we found him and Joy told him she worked at NBC, he promised to try to pan the camera over our way and get us in a shot.

Well, for the rest of the game we had to watch the plays plus watch for the camera to pan over to our section at which point I would stand up and hold the sign high above my head. All of those fans around us would yell, "Hold it up! The camera is pointing in our direction!" We all wanted to get on TV so those watching at home could see us and get green with envy that we were actually at the game and especially when we were blowing the other team completely out of the water! I laugh now at how funny we must have appeared as we struggled to get that sign out from under the seat and hurriedly thrusted it high into the air! Of course, all of us were convinced that we must have been seen by the camera at least one time!

We arrived home that evening completely exhausted but thrilled to have had that experience. And even when everyone told us we were nowhere to be seen on television, we were not disappointed, for we had shared an afternoon that nothing could dampen — nothing at all! It would serve as another rainbow, for the Lord had sent many our way over the last few years. We know His promises are sure! We had made another memory!

I'm always saying to Sandy, and to the girls I worked with at NBC, "Okay, girls, let's make a memory!" They look at me like I am crazy and say, "Oh, no! Here we go again!"

You see, when you live with cancer you come to realize the truth for us all — that none of us is promised any tomorrows. It is just so much more real for me. My time frame for life is limited so much more than those who do not live as I do. As Christians we should live that way every day, but we do not. I did not live that way before I developed cancer. Therefore, every chance I get now, I want to make those memories with my friends and loved ones because I will not have another chance. Through my "make a memory" philosophy, I hope to encourage them to take the time to make precious memories with each other after God calls me home.

Chapter 3

The Waiting Game

In mid-November, I accompanied Joy to her chemotherapy session. I mentioned to the oncology nurse that the injections I was giving Joy (three times a week) were extremely painful for her. The previous evening she had cried so hard after the injection that it had scared me. "I can't take it anymore! You'll never know how painful these injections are!" she screamed. Then she laid her head down and we both cried. I knew with all she had been through without complaint that this must truly be excruciating for her.

The nurse ordered some Lidocaine ointment for her. It was to be applied to the injection site one hour before giving the injection, to numb the area. We tried the cream the next day and, although it didn't take the pain away completely, it made the injections tolerable, and for that I thanked God.

Joy also had met with her doctor and it was decided that he would not attempt to drain the fluid around her left lung at this time. There was too much of a chance that cancer cells coming through the needle used to drain the fluid would invade the wall of her lung and we didn't want that to happen. He gave her more antibiotics and medication to suppress the still ever present cough. So far, that seemed to be working. I thanked God for the wisdom of her doctors. She was truly blessed to have such competent and caring people working with her. She always seemed to be comfortable with their decisions and confident that they were doing the best for her. Here once again I am amazed at God's perfect timing — the people that have been placed in Joy's life at the exact time she needed them. I am amazed and yet I don't know why when everything connected with her situation has been amazing.

Once again, the cancer was playing a waiting game with us but we would not wait and twiddle our thumbs! No! There were more memories to be made, more lessons to be learned, more work to be done for our Lord. No! Joy would not waste any of the time God gives her for He promises:

> *"But seek ye first His kingdom and His righteousness, and all these things will be given to you as well. Therefore do not worry about tomorrow, for tomorrow will worry about itself. Each day has enough trouble of its own."* — Matthew 7:33, 34

Joy knew she may only have today — I knew that could be true of me also.

"Lord, I guess it seems like a silly prayer to pray for something to lessen the pain of that shot, but I just can't take that anymore! The bone pain is so much greater, I know, but that seems to pale in comparison to the pain I suffer from that dumb injection! Is there anything you can do? I know Sandy is having a very difficult time giving it because the pain for me is so great."

I prayed that prayer several times and left it with the Lord. It seemed so silly in light of my other requests. And just then He answered as only He can. An ointment was provided by the doctor to take away the intense pain. It numbed the site of the injection and it really helped. I counted that as one of my best blessings. God supplied even my silliest of requests. Isn't He just wonderful!! I am learning to wait upon Him for everything — He will respond!

Chapter 4

His Strength Is Perfect

In spite of everything, including Joy's chemotherapy each week and, the bane of my existence, those hated injections, the holidays came and went, blessed as usual, and with that 1995 drew to a close and the dawning of a new year was upon us. What would 1996 bring? There had been no change in Joy's condition, no worsening of her cancer. Things were copacetic! We just praised God for yet another year.

February, and another trip to the doctor revealed much more lung fluid. The tap was still considered too dangerous and it was decided to try a different kind of chemotherapy.

"Is there a type of chemotherapy we could try that would not cause me to lose my hair?" Joy asked the doctor with hope in her voice.

"Well," he paused while thinking through his answer, "in fact there is a chemotherapy called Navelbine but it has other side effects such as neurological problems among others."

"Okay," she promptly stated, having already made up her mind even before he had time to get her the information on the possible side effects of the medication. "That is what I want. I can handle most any side effect and if I can at least keep my hair, I'm happy!"

"You win," the doctor said with a twinkle in his eyes. "You always run your own program anyway. I don't know why I don't hand you your chart and let you write my notes! Navelbine it is. But we will keep an eye on that lung." With that he laughed and shook his head again in disbelief at her vivaciousness and spirit in the face of yet another failed chemotherapy attempt. God's strength was present and so apparently at work in her life. She jumped off the table and we were on to bigger and better things. She handed me the information sheet on the new medication without even glancing at it, and told me to keep it or throw it away! She would keep her hair, at least for the present, and that was all that mattered. I prayed that the other side effects would not be too horrific! With her hair, Joy could still look "normal" even if she felt ill. At least she could shield herself from the pity that always followed her hair loss. And since she was still a master at disguising her pain, most of the time she appeared "normal"to the world. That was her desire.

Another CAT scan performed in March and it was still the consensus that a lung tap was not advisable. Her condition remained the same — no better, no worse. We accepted that and, as usual, Joy was content, reminding me once again that His strength is, and continues to be, perfect!

But he said to me, "My grace is sufficient for you, for my power is made perfect in weakness." Therefore I will boast all the more gladly about my weaknesses, so that Christ's power may rest on me. That is why, for Christ's sake, I delight in weaknesses, in insults, in hardships, in persecutions, in difficulties. For when I am weak, then I am strong. — 2 Corinthians 12:9-10

Dr. Roy Beveridge is one in a million! He was God's choice for me from the beginning; of that I am certain. He is a family man who truly cares about all of his patients, even the ones who are very stubborn and headstrong like I am. He treats his patients with respect and dignity. I have always felt that. I don't think he fully understands my relationship with the Lord, but I tell Him that God is really THE **Great Physician** even though I consider him to be a great physician! I think he gets my drift!

When he asks me a question that I sorta dance around without actually telling him the whole truth because I know of the consequences, he usually looks to Sandy (who is usually with me, and eager to rat on me), knowing that with her, he can get the full story! I'm really glad that she (and Jim also) trust him and have a good rapport with him as well. He has always included them in consultations and makes them a part of my whole treatment. Even though they do "rat" on me, I know all of them are working together for my best interest.

"Thank you, Lord, for Doctor Beveridge, Sandy, and Jim. We are a team and with you in charge, it is the best."

Chapter 5

A New Daughter

The winter of 1995-96 had been very severe and it seemed as though it would never end. When it eventually melted into spring with new life evident everywhere, we were reminded of God's marvelous creation and the promise of new opportunities to serve the creator. His power had been shown in the massive snowstorms that had blanketed the east coast and now it was seen again in the delicate, beautiful dogwood trees and magnificent azaleas that were prolific in the beautiful Commonwealth of Virginia.

With the glorious spring, came the announcement from our younger son, Adam, that he and Rita were engaged. We were all thrilled beyond words — we loved Rita! God was going to give us a new "daughter" and He couldn't have chosen a more wonderful girl! I was especially happy that Rita had become such good friends with our first darling "daughter," Julie. They truly love each other. Since both of our sons, Andrew and Adam, are very close, it was important to me that their wives develop a closeness as well. Now the four of them would be good friends. I thanked the Father. The wedding date would be June 7, 1997. It seemed like a long way off, but with all there was to do, I knew the time would fly by.

A wedding and the hope of a new daughter were very thrilling for my husband Jim and me. Julie had been such a blessing to us and we were so happy that she would soon have another "sister." Rita comes from a large family that loves the Lord. We looked forward to being joined together with them through the union of our children.

Joy invited Rita to move in with her until the marriage and Rita's parents were just thrilled. Rita had lived all of her life in a small rural community outside of Richmond, Virginia. The Northern Virginia area could be overwhelming to a small town girl and it was comforting to Rita's family to know we would take care of their little girl!

It was also during this spring that Rita and Adam graduated from Longwood College. It didn't seem possible that four years had passed since that first day of painful separation when I realized that our younger son was making a life of his own and I couldn't be there with him to smooth away the rough edges, kiss away the tears that were sure to come, and soothe the hurts. It is a process that all parents must go through, but we had survived in great shape. As we watched Adam on the podium leading his class in their alma mater, my eyes filled with tears. His father put his arm around my waist, silently reminding me of the pride that he, too, felt at that glorious moment. God is so faithful. He had led us through a very dark valley during Adam's first year of college, but now here was proof of His faithfulness once again.

And there beside us standing proudly were Adam's grandmother (his "Nina"), and Joy. Neither of them thought they would live to see this day and here they were with us to celebrate together as a family. "Great is thy faithfulness, Oh God, my Father. There is no shadow of turning with thee," as goes the famous hymn.

Hearing the news of Adam and Rita's wedding plans really gave me something to look forward to — something to think about instead of cancer! I love Rita and I was sure she was God's choice for Adam.

I had been alone for the first time in my life after my mom died in 1993, and so I took the opportunity to have a roommate by inviting Rita to live with me for the year before she and Adam were married. She wanted to move up to the Northern Virginia area after they graduated from college if she could get a job. That way with her job and Adam preparing for his career by substitute teaching until a permanent teaching job became available, they could save up some money for a whole year. I thought that sounded like a very mature thing to do. However, her parents were concerned about her being on her own for the first time in this huge metropolitan area. When I asked Rita about rooming with me and she told her parents, they were happy and relieved.

That year was very special to me. Rita and I became very close — she became like the little sister I never had. I will never forget it. I missed her very much when she moved out after the wedding, but I thank God for her and for the memories we shared. She will make a wonderful wife for Adam.

Chapter 6

Renewing My Spirit

Even though the spring had been filled with graduation and wedding plans to think about, it was also during these few months that I believe I was at my lowest ebb, emotionally! I was beginning to feel drained, trapped and smothered — too many people were depending on me. I realized that I, too, have a breaking point. And as much as I tried to pretend that I was strong and could do it all, I began to admit to myself that I could not. I was becoming angry at my situation and yet I really didn't want to be anywhere else. I didn't know what I wanted.

How confusing! I prayed and Jim and I discussed ways that I could cope. He is my sounding board and I'm afraid I sounded *loud and clear!* I had to change my attitude, I just had to. Rather, the Lord had to change it for me!

My mother's panic attacks were worsening and becoming more frequent; Joy seemed more dependent than ever because she longed to make the most of the time she had, and I understood that. She wanted to go on lots of day trips and she spent money well beyond reason, although not always on herself. She seemed more determined than ever to stay normal, whatever that is. I wanted to make the most of the time God was granting her. I wanted the time to be filled with wonderful memories; however, meeting everyone's needs seemed to be more and more difficult. Trying to fix everything for everybody was impossible and I was struggling. It is a struggle that every "fixer" knows well. I still have not fully learned my lesson very well. At times I know when to step back and at other times I am blinded by my desire to — yes — control the situation!

I was tired. I needed a rest. I needed to find a juniper tree as Elijah did in 1 Kings 19:5-8. The most frightening thing of all was that our small church was getting even smaller. I realized that the reason I felt like I did was not physical so much as it was spiritual. I needed a spiritual renewal for my soul. I was dying spiritually. I loved our congregation; but I longed once again to be a part of a growing church.

Because of the dwindling numbers, we had a very limited music program and I really missed that aspect of worship. Music has always been such an integral part of my life — to have little or no music was devastating to my soul. I wanted to be a part of a vibrant musical ministry because of the tremendous stress I was experiencing in my life. Jim needed to have a spiritual renewal as well. We needed refreshment that we were lacking. We had many discussions on the subject, but because of the love we felt for our church family, we stayed. However, after prayerful consideration, it was decided that the time had come for us to begin our search for another group of believers — another church.

Do you realize what a painful decision that was to be for us? Jim had grown up in that church from boyhood. We had met, married and had our children dedicated to the Lord there. We had served there in many capacities for over forty years; it was all that we had ever known, and we were now searching for another family. I believe it was one of the hardest decisions we have ever had to make as a couple — it broke my heart. And yet, I knew that unless we did something quickly, I would not make it — we had to feel spiritually healthy again. We had discussed this also with Adam and with Joy. Adam would be home again and he needed to have Christian friends his own age and a Bible study suited for young adults. He needed to be able to use the musical talents that God had given to him. Joy had been saying for some time that with her physical condition, she knew she, too, needed a spiritual infusion. She knew that it was imperative that she make a move — we just all wanted to be in church together as we had been for so long.

Andrew and Julie had for some time been attending a sound evangelical church and were already involved in a Sunday School class and a Bible study; but as much as we loved their church, it was just too large a congregation for us and too far away from our home to allow us to actively participate in membership. They were concerned about us and were praying for us.

God worked in a most unexpected way. I called our cousin, Scott, one day in February to get his mother's address because I wanted to send flowers to her home upon the death of Scott's father. We hadn't talked in a while, so we used the opportunity to catch up on our families' news. In the course of our conversation I inquired as to where they were attending church. Scott told us they were involved in Faith Evangelical Presbyterian Church. The congregation was then meeting in a nearby local school building. I shared with him more about our situation, some of which he had known about for some time, and he invited us to visit Faith the following Sunday.

My words cannot adequately explain to you the joy I felt in my heart during that wonderful service. I had prayed before we had made arrangements to attend that during our search (which we anticipated would be a long and difficult one) the Lord would go before us and reveal His will to us. I know that the Lord led us to Faith, and that He led us there first because He knew we needed a renewal quickly. I just didn't realize that our new church home was to be the first church we attended!

I thought about the sermon all week long, and I sang worship and praise songs over and over in my soul! We were impressed by the warm congregation and their obvious love for the Lord. My whole attitude was changed that week. I could hardly wait to go back. However, Jim and I had to agree on this decision, and it couldn't be made lightly. He, too, was very much comforted by the spirit that we felt there. But we needed much more information before we could make a decision. Jim was very involved in the leadership of our church as he had been for many years. I knew this decision, any decision to leave, would prove to be very difficult. We invited the pastor, Dr. W. Graham Smith, over to our home and asked him to share with us as well as with our Julie, and Joy, the doctrine of the church and its statements of faith. We knew we had to be very careful in our decision. We were pleased to learn that with the exception of the modes of baptism and communion, our beliefs were the same — the essentials, the precious essentials, were all there! It was the same as our dear Grace Brethren. The pastor was loving and caring and assured us that he would be praying for us as we sought God's will for us. He was clearly touched by our concerns.

After prayerful consideration and much discussion, we all decided that this was where the Lord was leading us. We had dinner with our pastor and his wonderful wife not too many weeks later and told them of our decision. I had prayed for their understanding. Thankfully, they were most loving and supportive. They, too, recognized the limitations of our church and they were praying also for God's leading in their own lives as well. Jim and I agreed that our last Sunday would be May 19, 1996. The pastor asked that we allow him to read our resignation letter to the church board. Soon thereafter he would read his own letter to them. It was the end of a chapter in all our lives. We had grown and would continue to grow and I realized that growth is sometimes very painful — only time would heal! How we had come to love all those we were leaving and how much of God's Word we had learned over our many years there! We would be eternally grateful to God for those blessings.

It would take much more time at our new church before we would know if the Lord would have this be our home; we would attend their new members' class and learn much more about the congregation and the church. But for now, we were content to worship and receive spiritual nourishment and let the Lord bathe us in His peace and love. It proved to be only a short time before we would feel very much at home!

I don't think I can last another Sunday unless I get a spiritual uplift, Lord. I need guidance, wisdom, encouragement from your Word. I need to hear God speak to me. I don't want to go to church anymore just because I love the people, or because I feel comfortable.

Sandy, Jim and I had talked about it for some time and I know they feel as I do but they are so very involved there and they have been for over forty years! I knew they were having a struggle with it. But even if it meant leaving them in order to find something more for my needy spirit, I knew I had to.

Then Sandy and Jim visited a new church soon after that and told us of the spirit there and of the wonderful sermon they had heard. She repeated it as she had heard it and I knew she had been blessed. Adam and I visited the next Sunday.

Praise God for a little Irish man, Pastor Graham Smith. His sermon spoke straight to my heart that Sunday morning. I needed to know that through everything that was going on in my life, God cared — I didn't have to do it alone — I could give up my independence and lean totally on Him. I always knew that, but I needed to *hear* it and to have it reinforced to me over and over again as cancer ripped through my body.

The people were genuine and caring, like at Grace, only more of them! The music, which we had missed for so long, ministered to my heart. That very Sunday I knew God wanted me there. I prayed that the Rices would feel that way too, but I had to do this for myself, now! Even if it meant doing it without them, hard as that would be, I had to! Little did I know how many blessings would follow as I made that decision!

Chapter 7

Kindred Spirits

It was on Sunday evening, April 21, that I discovered a small lump in my right breast! I kept poking at it all evening hoping that it would prove to be my imagination. Joy's cancer had begun in her right breast. It must just be a coincidence, a sympathy pang, anything but a lump! However, each time I felt for it, it was there. No! I knew it was definitely a lump. It was very small, but nevertheless it was a lump.

I told Jim about it and he, too, was able to feel it on the outer side of my right breast. I decided to call my private physician the very next morning.

I didn't sleep very well that night. Each time I awoke I would feel for the lump and each time it was still there! Joy's whole experience began racing through my mind. If this proved to be cancer, could I handle it as she had? What would I tell my children? How would they handle it? How could I possibly tell Jim, my mother, or Joy? I wanted to see Rita and Adam marry, I wanted grandchildren, I wanted to grow old with Jim, I wanted ... How could I handle the disappointment of not being able to witness all of that in my lifetime? How gracious would I be in the face of death? How would it affect my own witness, if it proved to be cancer? I found it difficult to pray so I closed my eyes and spent a restless night.

My doctor confirmed in his office the following morning that he also felt a small lump. At least I wasn't imagining it, as if that were a consolation!

I was to have a mammogram that afternoon. My supervising nurse, Harriet, is not only a terrific person to work for, but she has been a wonderful friend as well. She insisted on driving me quite a distance to pick up my previous mammograms and accompany me to my appointment. I never asked Harriet to do that. She called my doctor's office, found out what I had to do, and the next thing I knew I was in her car. It was an answer to prayer for me. Jim had an appearance in court that morning and I had assured him that I would be fine. I knew he would have canceled everything if I wanted him to go with me, but I really didn't want to do that. I didn't want anyone else to panic. I wanted to remain calm. After all, there wasn't anything to panic about, yet. Then why was my heart feeling so unsettled?

I had wanted to avoid telling Joy because I knew it would bring up such painful memories for her, but I also knew that not to tell her would bring serious repercussions for me! Not too surprisingly, she was waiting at the doctor's office for me and Harriet when we arrived.

After waiting for what seemed like an age, I had a mammogram and then a sonogram. Both proved to be negative, Praise God! The small "lump" appeared to be only a part of my bone structure on that side of my breast. I would need close follow-up for the next year by a specialist but at least for the time being, the "lump" appeared normal for me. I immediately called Jim as I had promised.

Joy was obviously very relieved, as was Harriet. Their presence with me made me realize how very fortunate people are who have support during these times in our lives. How very important it is to be ready and willing to be there for someone who is hurting. I saw my role in Joy's life through my own need and I have never been more aware of its importance. I would continue to be there for her because I knew now, firsthand, how very needed it was.

This crisis passed quickly but I had been able, in a very small way, to taste of the years past and I didn't like it. The taste was very bitter and I thanked God that it was not my portion, at least not for now. I only know that God will continue to give to me, as He has in the past, the same grace and strength that He has so graciously given to Joy, if and when I need it to face any situation! But I couldn't help wonder if I could face it as graciously as she has. Would I have her same courage and spirit? For a while during this short period of time which seemed like an eternity, I seriously questioned whether or not I could. I needed to remember that for now I didn't need the bridge for I had not yet come to that river.

While waiting for Sandy, a million things were going through my head. "Lord, for the first time, I question you. I don't want her to have to go through what I've been going through for years! Why, Lord, would this happen?"

I tried to hold back my tears but I just couldn't. I wanted to have her protected from the stares, the sickness, the pain. I cried over and over to my Father to please let it not be. If I could take what might be hers and add it to mine then I asked Him to allow me to bear her cross. I love her that much.

"She has a family and they need her, Lord. I need her!"

Oh, what a mighty God we serve! The tests proved negative! For now she would not have to bear that cross. "Thank you, Father. Thank you so much. I love you."

Chapter 8

God Knows The "Why"

Just as things were getting back to "normal" and the 1996 summer vacation was around the corner, I was personally faced with another completely unexpected health concern.

For two days I had been experiencing pain just below my right shoulder blade. Why wouldn't it go away? Vacation was quickly approaching and the end of the school year was always very hectic trying to close my clinic for the summer. I didn't need this!

On June 10, Joy was to begin taking a new IV medication called Arridia which was supposed to strengthen her weakened bones. It was her choice and against the nurses' advice to take her first treatment on the same day she was to take chemotherapy. I thought that was just too much medication for one day, but you know Joy! She wanted to get it all over with on one day so she could — you know — be normal again. She just couldn't afford to lose two days out of her life!

Joy left the doctor's office right after her treatment and, despite feeling extremely wiped out, she went to work. Her supervisor called me on that early June morning and was very concerned about Joy. She told me Joy could barely walk and wanted to do nothing but sleep, very much unlike her! Everyone at her office had panicked. I assured her that I would call the doctor's office right away and get back to her. Until then I asked that they just let her sleep and keep an eye on her.

I phoned the doctor's office and her nurse told me that the reaction was probably very normal considering Joy's most unwise decision to take a combination of the two medications on the same day! But she knew all too well that telling Joy, "No, you cannot do

47

that," falls on deaf ears, and it is often better to just let her find out for herself because sometimes, just sometimes, she will amaze you at her stamina even in the midst of her weakened condition. The doctor and his staff had learned that a long time ago!

I called NBC and requested that someone in the office drive Joy home. I checked on her throughout the remainder of the day. Needless to say, she began taking the monthly four-hour Arridia treatment on a different day than her weekly chemotherapy session. She had, albeit reluctantly, accepted the fact that once a month she had to give up two days instead of one, for her health!

The following day, June 11, Joy was back to work and feeling pretty good, but the pain had worsened in my shoulder blade, so much so that I slept very little that night and was in agony by early dawn, June 12. I sat by the phone and waited for an appropriate time to call Kathy, the wonderful office manager in my doctor's office. She had given me specific instructions to call her at home any time day or night if I needed to see the doctor. I appreciated that offer, but pre-dawn seemed unreasonable unless I felt near death! I was close!

Kathy told me to be at the office right at 9:00 unless I felt I needed to go to the emergency room. I wanted to try to avoid that, so I told her I would be at the office at 9:00. I struggled with help from Jim to get dressed and get to the office. Upon examination, it was decided that I needed to go to the emergency room of our local hospital, where a lung scan revealed a blood clot in my right lung.

Once again, all too soon, I found myself facing the possibility of a shortened life. Thoughts raced through my mind as I held tightly onto Jim's hand. Rita, so sweet, was to become my "daughter" next year and maybe I would not be there to see that. Maybe I wouldn't live to see Julie and Rita give us grandchildren. That same feeling that I had when I had gone through the experience with the breast cancer scare only two months previous was pressing upon me, only this time I feared imminent death. A blood clot can move at any time!

I know now a little of what Joy says when she talks about complete dependence upon God! Losing yourself to Him completely because you know that only He can give you the strength

48

that you so desperately need in the face of death! I called upon Him and asked for that strength. I was at the edge of the river now and I needed the bridge. Jim and I had reared two wonderful sons and they had both found wonderful mates. My life had been rich and full of God's blessings. Our marriage, our family, our friends — I had been given more than most people ever have so how could I ask for more even though I so much wanted more!

Heparin was begun through IV to dissolve the blood clot and medication was given to try to alleviate the severe pain still cutting through my back like a dagger! Nothing worked to quiet the pain; not even Demerol or morphine put a dent in it. Sleep was nonexistent! I was therefore completely exhausted from sleep deprivation and the continual severe pain. I prayed for something to work.

The following day, an angiogram revealed no clot despite the lung scan result! I was given a pain medication in the form of a patch used for people in severe pain as a result of cancer. That almost immediately alleviated the pain. I was discharged from the hospital four days later greatly relieved that the "clot" was gone and that the intense pain was greatly reduced.

It remains unclear to this day as to why a blood clot was clearly revealed and then a further test performed two days later showed no clot. Perhaps God allowed this so that I could focus my life ... and focus I did! Maybe I needed to see just a glimpse of that bridge that Joy talks about when she says, "God doesn't build a bridge until we get to the river," to see that God's strength is appropriated to us all no matter how wide or narrow the river.

No explanation has been offered as to the cause of the severe pain, and to this day that area has been pain free! I have read since then that estrogen therapy has been found to cause clots in women's legs and lungs. My physician reduced my estrogen dosage when I was released from the hospital.

Whatever the explanation, God allowed me to go through that experience for a purpose. One of Joy's favorite expressions lately has been, "God knows the 'Why.'" I may not know His full purpose for it for a long time or not even in my lifetime; however, I do know that "... *in all things God works for the good of those who love him, who have been called according to his purpose"* (Romans 8:28). And the same strength He has given to Joy these past few years had been available to me just when I needed it and I knew He would continue to provide. He is all sufficient! He supplied the bridge when I came to the river and He carried me across!

I was looking forward to summer vacation more than anything. God had given me more of them than I ever thought I would have, and for that I was very grateful.

June 10 was my first dose of Arridia which will strengthen my bones and hopefully protect them from the cancer. I wanted to take the Arridia and the chemo on the same day because I just hate to miss work because of too many appointments. I thought it was a good thing to do although the nurse told it me was a mistake. My body — my decision. Who knows better than I do about what I can take? Right?

I went to work when I finished at the doctor's office. By the time I got to my office it was all I could do to reach the sofa. I have never felt so much pain! I felt like I had been hit with a Mack truck. I prayed silently for strength to help me withstand the pain. My supervisor called Sandy at work so she could call the doctor for me.

Praise God it was a normal reaction for someone who would be so crazy as to take both Arridia and chemo on the same day. Maybe I don't know as much about my body as I thought I did!

God made me realize that I wanted to do things my way even down to my treatments. He showed me that I could not. It's one day at a time ... no rushing ... no jumping ahead ... no heroics. I must be still and know that He is God and He is in charge and has placed nurses and doctors in my life for my good and His glory. It had been a hard lesson to learn.

And then, the unexpected! I couldn't believe that Sandy was in the hospital. Jim called me early on June 12 and told me they suspected a clot in her lung! I prayed and asked God to give the doctors wisdom and to give her peace. I prayed for Jim, Nina (Sandy's mom), and the boys as well. I prayed for me, too. It had only been two months since we had faced her breast cancer scare. What was happening, Lord?

We faced it together during those few days, her family and I. It was difficult because the doctors couldn't seem to find anything

51

to help with the pain. I knew only too well that feeling! I cried my eyes out each night and kept the Lord busy with my prayers.

We praised Him once again when the crisis was finally over and she was home. It had been a very trying time for all of us but we were going to get to go on vacation together and that cheered us all up. Everything just seemed to be great when we were all at the beach!

"Lord, thank you for healing Sandy. I know you sent her to help me through my cancer, and I need her so much ... flesh and blood just feels so good sometimes, even though I know you are there ... really I do!"

Chapter 9

The Bear

Summer vacation was great even though I had to use a part of it to recuperate. I was glad to get to go to the beach, and I realized that for five years in a row Joy had had to face the possibility of not getting to go with us because of her health. Only then did I understand the feeling of disappointment that would have caused. The possibility of losing something always tends to make us see more clearly how dear that "something" is! For the rest of the summer, Joy's condition remained stationary. Her chemotherapy continued and she still had hair. Praise God!

Just before the end of the summer, Jim and I took our darling, then eleven-year-old niece, Amber, and my mother to the mountain for one last summer picnic before school started.

Jim had been kidding Amber the whole weekend about seeing a bear (that being a remote possibility). She was thrilled with the anticipation of seeing a bear and also with assurance from us, of seeing deer, for we have never failed to see them at our favorite picnic area on Skyline Drive near our mountain home. We had planned to go there the evening before we were to come home, eventide being the best time to see the most deer. Jim kept talking about the black bear all the way to Elk Wallow.

As we entered the picnic area, the deer were out in force to greet us. What a wonderful sight for Amber to see! Because it was late in the afternoon and most people had perhaps had their fill of summer picnics, the park was practically empty. Amber was ecstatic as we selected an ideal picnic spot and carried our basket to the table. She was so excited about feeding the deer that she could hardly eat.

We hadn't been there very long until we noticed a man several yards away with a video camera pointed up into a tree. The deer around our table stopped, perked up their ears and immediately scampered off just as we saw the man with the camera. We sensed that he wasn't videotaping birds or squirrels. It was something big!

Amber, of course, wanted to check out the situation and she started off towards the man with the camera. I decided she couldn't go alone so, with Jim keeping Mom company, I trailed off after her.

She had reached the "video spot" and was looking up to the top of a huge tree. Suddenly she whirled around and came running towards me.

"Aunt Sandy, there is a bear up in that tree and that man over there is taking pictures of him. A bear," she whispered ever so *loudly*, "A BEAR! Uncle Jim said I'd see a bear."

I had trouble believing it was a bear because that was so unlikely. "Oh, Amber," I said, sounding very skeptical but not wanting her to be disappointed. "I don't think it is really a bear!"

"Aunt Sandy," she said very matter-of-factly, and somewhat annoyed at my skepticism, "I saw it and it is a bear. If that isn't a bear, then I'm blind," she whispered loudly while pointing up into the tree!

At that statement she pulled my hand and crept closer to the tree and the man videotaping the "bear." Sure enough, as my eyes focused up the tree I could see a rather large fuzzy-looking black object that was most definitely a bear!

The man with the video camera quietly told us that he and his family saw the bear cub scamper past them and climb up the tree. The baby had apparently been separated from his mother because the man told us that he looked thin for his size and appeared confused. As we all gazed up into the tree at the frightened cub, Amber was absolutely mesmerized.

Just about that time, my mother decided she, too, wanted to see the bear. As she got up from the picnic table and before Jim could come around to help her, she turned around and fell to the ground. Amber, glancing up that way to motion her grandmother

54

and Uncle Jim to come see the bear, saw her grandmother fall. She grabbed my hand and we raced up to the table. I knew mother was in a great deal of pain and I was certain she had broken her hip or her leg. Jim and I carefully helped her up while supporting her hip and leg.

I knew Jim could not get our station wagon up the incline to get her. I also knew it would be impossible for us to carry her down the hill without perhaps further injuring her leg.

Just then the man that was using the video camera saw what had happened, and he and his son came to help us. The cameraman was a local minister and his son happened to own a sport utility vehicle and offered to drive it up the incline so that we could get Mother down the hill to our car and to the local hospital. God had provided that help and I marveled once again at His perfect timing. The park was completely empty with the exception of two families; one of those families needed the other one who had exactly what was needed! And further, both families were themselves in the same family, the Family of God! It would be only the first of His blessings during this crisis in our lives.

We got mother into the station wagon and lowered the front seat so that she was practically lying flat. The trip to the hospital took about twenty minutes. Amber, bless her heart, held her grandmother's hand and I silently prayed that Mother would not go into shock before we could get help for her.

Once at the emergency room, Mother was immediately cared for and given pain medication. Her hip was x-rayed and indeed it was found to be broken! The night turned out to be very long and very stressful for us all. It was then 7:00 in the evening. There was no orthopedic surgeon on duty nor would there be until Monday morning, three days away, and my mother needed immediate surgery! We needed a transport team to take her by ambulance to Alexandria, two hours away. Their only transport team had just left for Martinsburg, West Virginia, and would not be returning until at least midnight or later!

Mother was getting more and more confused with the pain medication and we didn't know what to do. We considered taking her home in our car but it was determined that she was in no shape for us to transport her ourselves for she needed to have medical assistance with her on the trip. We were considering a private transport team at a cost of approximately $1000 because we thought we had no alternative! I could hear the staff on the telephone and talking amongst themselves trying to think of every available thing they could in order to expedite our trip at the most reasonable cost to us.

At some point in the evening I looked up to see the young man who had used his truck to help my mother at the park. He and his wife and baby stopped by the emergency room to check on Mom. She did recognize him and as he held her hand and told her they were praying for her, I thanked God once again for His faithfulness.

It was shortly after that visit that we were informed by the doctor on duty that they had been able to contact their transport team and they had gotten a nurse who said she would ride with them. They would gladly take us to Alexandria after they returned from Martinsburg. It would be a turnaround trip for the driver, but he was willing. Praise God!

It would be 5:00 the next morning before I would get Mom settled in her bed at our local hospital and Jim, Amber and I would fall into bed for a couple of hours. It was only the beginning of a very long ordeal.

My mother had her surgery the following day and was put back into her own room just hours afterwards. We thought this was a very good sign. However, the next day she began having chest pain. After it was determined that she had suffered a mild heart attack, she was moved into the cardiac care unit. For almost a week she would be there hovering between life and death. Her blood pressure would drop very low and she would hallucinate. Her doctor talked to us about a "No Code" (do not resuscitate) on Mother and, through tears, my sister, Carolyn, and I agreed it was the best thing to do.

We took turns visiting her in the unit as we prayed, cried and waited to see what the Lord's will was to be. One particular evening as she seemed to be slipping further and further away, I put a tape on the tape player that we had been allowed to take into the intensive care unit. While listening to that beautiful chorus, "I Exalt

Thee, Oh Lord," and with tears flowing down my cheeks, I began to beg the Lord to give me more time with my mother even though He had already given her over ninety years. The last few of those ninety years had not been easy on either of us as we tried to make sense of the aging process that is sometimes accompanied by things that you don't expect, like depression, dementia and role-reversal. Depression had been consuming my mother until I didn't know her. And what I did know, I fought and resisted until I had become bitter and angry. I didn't like being the mother. I didn't like it one bit. Couple that with the stress and pain of seeing Joy's deterioration from cancer while caring for her for the past six years and I cried for myself, as well as for Mom. I couldn't have my mother die and live with this pain in my heart and with the knowledge that I hadn't really tried my best to understand her depression and had allowed her to fight it almost alone for the past two years.

I began to bargain with God, something I thought I would never do! But then, I had never experienced this type of pain before. In the coming weeks I would need God's strength again and again as well as His mercy, wisdom and forgiveness.

It would be a long time before I fully understood what the Psalmist meant when he said, *"It was good for me to be afflicted so that I might learn your decrees"* (Psalm 119:71). Adversity teaches valuable lessons but the lessons are often very painful — very, very painful!

Our souls represent some kind of battlefield if we belong to the Lord. The point is whether or not we hang in there and fight as Job did. And of course, if we are trusting in the Lord to be our Captain, we cannot lose.

Sandy and Jim had faced one battle after another in rapid succession. They will be victorious in this I know, but it hurt my heart to see them have to go through the fire once again. I pray for Nina each night and for all of "my family" as they go through this. "Lord, help me to have the strength to help them in any way that I can!"

Chapter 10

Tribulation Bringeth Patience

Indeed it is a hard lesson to learn — the lesson of patience. I had stopped praying for it! You see, His Word says, "Tribulation bringeth patience." Wisdom? Yes. Knowledge? Yes, I prayed for those. But never for patience! Of course, I grew in the Lord during those times of tribulation. This particular crisis proved to be no exception, but I certainly did not like the process.

My mother's condition became stable and she was able to be taken out of the intensive care unit and placed into her own room. Her hallucinations continued and she wasn't eating very well, but we knew she was better. Our dear Pastor Graham Smith visited her often and prayed with her. How she loved him! His presence seemed to bring peace to her heart. Even though she couldn't remember many of the visitors she received, she always remembered when he had been there. We thanked God once again for leading us to our new church and the wonderful family we had found there.

Mother's doctor discharged her after another week and placed her into a rehabilitation center in order to teach her how to use her leg once again. This move proved to be rather traumatic for Mom at first. However, before too long she adjusted and after only two weeks, we were able to take her home.

The first few weeks at home were very trying for the whole family as we made physical adjustments in our home and dealt with the many emotional issues as well. Mother needed to be helped to the bathroom, have her meals served to her bed, and bathed and changed often during that time. We had help for her until I got home each afternoon so that I was able to start back to work. I thanked God for those wonderful friends who volunteered to help us with Mom's many needs.

Before too long, the nurses and physical therapists were satisfied that Mom could function pretty well on her own and they were discharged. I continued to help her with her exercises and she progressed very well. By Christmas, she was well enough to go to my sister's home for a couple of days, as she had done for a number of years.

God dealt with me very seriously during those long and sometimes lonely weeks, and I have never forgotten my promise to Him, even though I fail Him from time to time. It is still very difficult and I find myself short-tempered and grouchy at times. I realize that these are very normal feelings and I must stop beating myself over the head with guilt. Things would never be the same again. My mother would not be young again and be "my mother." I was the mother, and I had to accept that.

Even though my mother accepted the Lord long ago and she has assurance of eternal life, she had been, for some time, afraid to die. We had discussed it many times and I know it was something that had weighed heavily on her mind. She felt so guilty for being afraid. I have learned that many elderly people, Christians included, have that same fear. It's not so much dying as it is the fear of the unknown. As we get older, our thought processes are different. If we become childlike in our old age, and surely I know firsthand that we do, then we must place ourselves back into our childhood and remember that we were once afraid of many things, not the least being death. Therefore it would naturally follow that for a great many elderly people, especially those suffering from dementia and depression, death would be especially fearful.

Mother told me one day not long after coming home from the hospital, "You know, I thought I was going to die when I was in the hospital, but it was really all right because I know that when that happens, I will be in heaven with Jesus." Her experience helped her face that reality and, in turn, her acceptance of that has helped me also. There were still times when with her dementia, she forgot our many discussions about death and dying and her promise from God that He will never leave her, but I knew that God would bring that to her remembrance and would build that bridge when she came to that river. Remember, He never builds that bridge until we need it. He doesn't give us grace and strength to face any situation until it is necessary. We must depend upon Him to give it when it becomes necessary, and He will. He always does!

I thanked God for the extra time He allowed me to have with my mother even though times were still difficult, at best. My children needed to see me handle the situation with grace and strength. Up until then I honestly didn't think I had always done that.

I needed patience and I was afraid to pray for it. Not just patience towards my mother, but patience to sit still and wait upon the Lord. *"I waited patiently for the Lord; he turned to me and heard my cry. He gave me a firm place to stand. He put a new song in my mouth, a hymn of praise to our God. Many will see and fear and put their trust in the Lord"* (Psalm 40:1-3). It could be that the patience that I needed to pray for was patience to wait before I gave an answer to a seemingly ridiculous question posed to me by my mother. Or patience to wait before I reminded her harshly that the question she had just asked me I had answered a hundred times and afterwards having to watch the hurt in her eyes at my inexcusable behavior. Patience to wait upon an answer from the Lord before I gave my own answer. And the guilt! Oh, the guilt that I had to deal with afterwards — perhaps I wouldn't have had to face that any more if I had used God's answers.

So maybe, just maybe, I needed to be brave enough to pray for patience once again, a different kind of patience.

I'll never understand the elderly and their fear of dying because I'm not there. Of course, it is even harder for me because I know (well, I'm fairly sure, barring a miracle from my Lord) that I will never have the experience of being "elderly." I cannot judge, but for everyone I'm sure acceptance of death is different. I've had a lot of time to think about it. I guess the older you get, the more of life you want to experience if your life has been wonderful. Sandy and Jim had done everything possible to make Nina's life wonderful and she would agree that it had been just that ... wonderful. I guess in a way if I'm honest, I will admit that I would like to have had a chance to be "elderly." Maybe in a way I'm jealous of people who are.

But I know I wouldn't change who God has caused me to become and I have accepted His will for my life, however short it may be. Nina will be ready when God chooses to take her because He doesn't give us the grace to accept anything until we are faced with it. Until then, I believe He understands our fears even when we don't.

Chapter 11

Realizing A Dream

I had been trying for almost a year to get my first book published. I had started the book in 1993, just before Joy was to have her stem cell transplant. I was desperate for the world to learn of her courage and faith in the midst of her battle with cancer. Her story would give hope to the hopeless. I wanted the world to praise God for His mercy and for His goodness to us. The book was written as a tribute to my husband and my children for their support and love to me and to Joy during this time in our lives. It is titled *To Run The Race With Joy!*

Joy's contacts at NBC enabled us to get endorsements from Katie Couric and Willard Scott, two very prominent television personalities. I thanked God for their willingness to lend their names to my book. It certainly couldn't hurt my chances of getting the book published.

However, even with those great names, I never really in my heart of hearts thought the book would be published. I had written it so simply, so plainly, no "reading between the lines" to figure it out. I knew those who read it would marvel at Joy's story for one couldn't help but be inspired by that. But who would care about my life or my thoughts or, for that matter, my spiritual growth through the last few years? And yet, I had learned so much and had experienced so much of God's richest blessings that I needed to write it down whether or not anyone else read about it. And it was the only way I could write it because I had lived it too. I still continue to live it. Many other people find themselves in a similar role as a caregiver. Maybe they need to know that the same God who cares for and strengthens the afflicted they care for, loves them just as much and is there to strengthen them also.

And so, I wrote query letter after query letter to the leading publishing houses in the country and spent much money on postage and printing. I received many nice responses to my letters and much encouragement, but no takers.

I decided to join a Christian writers group and maybe get some new ideas on how to publish. Jim had assured me that we would self-publish if it became necessary. He had read my manuscript and greatly encouraged me as did several of my trusted and dearest friends. Perhaps, I thought, a writers group would be helpful. I asked Joy to accompany me and we went to our first meeting.

It was a dark, cool, rainy evening as we drove up to the church where the meetings were held. As we entered the room, I realized almost immediately that this was perhaps not a very wise decision. The room was very cold and my feet were freezing in a matter of minutes! We had to sit on hard chairs as we wrapped up in our coats!

The group consisted of four members plus Joy and me. The leader of the group had had several things published, her forte being Christian science fiction. She was obviously a very intelligent woman but seemed to possess no real warmth or people skills. One young woman was writing Christian romance novels and the remaining female was into poetry. The only male member of our group also wrote poetry.

We had a rather interesting and informative open discussion but I found it hard to concentrate because one of the women had brought her young son to the meeting and, oblivious to her, he proceeded to destroy an adjoining classroom where he had been placed during our meeting. I watched and listened as he ripped the mini blinds at the window of the room and managed to rearrange them into all sorts of interesting shapes and sizes, never again to be used for the purpose to which they were originally intended. Several times his mother glanced his way and gave him that "Please don't do that, honey" look. However, it was soon apparent from his continuation of the activity that perhaps I should suggest to his mother that she would do well to concentrate her efforts on finding the solution to his obvious "genetic" hearing and vision problems!

The leader of the group then asked the lone gentleman to read aloud a piece of poetry that he had written. Well, I was certainly glad that Joy and I did not have eye contact during his reading because we surely would have embarrassed ourselves to no end if we had. His poetry was about a pack of English hound dogs running down a hill barking in the night. Aside from that, I really don't know the meaning that was intended. The dogs were supposed to symbolize Satan and there were mentions of blood and darkness, and — well — you get the picture! The group sat in rapt attention (including, of course, Dennis the Menace's mother) with all eyes focused on the poet. I couldn't believe what he was reading. It made no sense to me at all! I never looked at Joy once and for very good reason. I knew she was as confused as I was, especially when everyone seemed to be enthralled with his reading and had rave reviews for him. I guess Joy and I are just too simple-minded to have understood the reading.

As we left the building after the meeting and were out of earshot of the group, we looked at each other and simultaneously said, "Ruff, ruff" as we doubled over in uproarious laughter.

"I was so afraid you would look at me," Joy said, as she wiped tears from her eyes.

"Yes," I said through giggles. "It would have been all over if we had made eye contact." Not that either one of us planned to go again, but we certainly didn't want to show our lack of literary appreciation! So we chalked that up to experience and continued looking for publishers on our own.

One day in August after one of Joy's weekly chemotherapy sessions, she seemed especially tired and so much weaker. We watched as she continued to lose weight and her stamina continued to wane. I became very concerned that perhaps if things continued the way they had been, Joy might not be around to see the book published. The thought of having it accepted when it was too late for her to see it was alarming.

So, I prayed about it for a while, got my *Christian Writer's Market Guide*, by Sally Stuart, and then opened it up to no particular page. As I scanned the page, my eyes fell on CSS Publishing Company, Lima, Ohio. I had never heard of them, but then they had not heard of me either so I decided rather than send a few chapters and a query letter, I would just call them.

"Hello. My name is Sandy Rice and I have just completed my first book about my best friend who has breast cancer. The title of the book is *To Run the Race with Joy*. I think it is pretty good and many people who have read it seem to think that also, so I wondered if you would be interested in it?" Didn't that sound professional?

The young lady who answered the phone asked me some questions about the book, foremost, was it written from a Christian standpoint. My reply to her: "Absolutely. Jesus Christ is on every page of my book."

"Well," she continued, "CSS doesn't usually publish that type of book. We are known for our children's publications and sermon helps for pastors and laymen. However, your book sounds very interesting, so why don't you send it to us and maybe someone will take a look at it."

I didn't really think much more about it. I had a couple more query letters out there so I decided to send CSS the entire manuscript at the suggestion of the receptionist I had spoken with, and just wait.

Approximately two weeks later Jim came home from work with our daily mail. In it was my self-addressed envelope from CSS and from the size of it I knew it contained my manuscript. "Looks like another rejection, honey," he said with a consoling look on his face.

Well, I had gotten plenty of them so this was just another one to add to the list. I slowly opened the package and was prepared to read the usual "I am sorry to inform you" letter. I couldn't believe my eyes when this letter began "We are pleased to inform you that our editorial staff has accepted your manuscript for publication ..." I cannot even tell you how excited I was as I read the words out loud for Jim and my mother to hear. The letter continued that their publication list was full for 1997 but they were making an exception and mine was be slated to be published in Spring 1997!

"I'm an author!" I screamed with excitement, literally bursting with joy. "I'm really an author. They are going to publish my book. They like my book!"

I opened up the manuscript, already edited, and went through it to find out how much they had cut and what changes they wanted in order to publish. I had prayed that whoever did take a chance on me and publish my book, would not cut anything out because it was my story and I didn't want any part of it cut. I knew that was a dream because all of the things I had ever read about publishing told me that it was a foregone conclusion that a manuscript would be cut, sometimes beyond recognition, especially since I was a first time author.

I praised God out loud as I scanned the manuscript. Nothing was changed. Nothing at all! Only a few punctuation markings and one or two sentences, but beyond that, nothing!

Words cannot describe my emotions, my praise, my heartbeat! It was a dream beyond anything I had ever hoped for. I knew then that it was God's will. Only God could have directed me to that page in the *Market Guide* and to CSS. Only He could have led CSS to read that particular manuscript and choose to publish it when they had never published that type of book before. Only God. Only God! I began making phone calls!

First of all, I want to say that I had no doubt at all that Sandy's book, our story, would be published! "In God's time," I would keep telling her. I knew her writing was so good, so easy to read and so much from her heart. But I don't think she believed me when I would tell her.

We had such fun trying to find a publisher, trying to decide which chapters to send in for review. Most of the time we agreed but I liked them all, so I usually just let Sandy decide. After all, she is the writer!

The day Sandy called me to tell me she had heard from a publisher that wanted our book, I cannot explain my feelings except to say that I have heard people say that at certain times in their lives when God answered their prayers they felt a tremendous burden had been lifted from their shoulders. Well, that is exactly what I felt like. I knew just then the "why" of my cancer. There and then, I thanked God for my cancer ... God would be glorified through me as He could be in no other way.

Chapter 12

A New Mission

I started making phone calls to everyone I knew to share the good news. First, of course, I called Joy who was on her way home.

"You're kidding," she said as I screamed the news into her ear. "You're not kidding!" she yelled back into the phone, her voice trembling with excitement. "You're not kidding?"

"No! I'm definitely not kidding," I said. I proceeded to read the letter to her so quickly because of my excitement, that I had to read it to her twice before she could understand my babblings!

"I'm coming right over!" she answered, hardly able to contain herself. "I have got to see it!"

I hung the phone up after reminding her to drive carefully because I knew she was far too excited to be exactly rational! I began making more phone calls. No one was home!! I called my sister, my sister-in-law, friends from church, my co-workers, neighbors — everyone I knew. And phone call after phone call, no one was at home. I was finally able to reach my supervising nurse, Harriet. I shared the news with her and she was very, very excited. More than that, she was overjoyed that I asked her to write a comment about my book (because she had already read the manuscript) so that I could include it in the final draft.

Harriet had truly become a friend to Joy and to me. She cared very much about Joy and Joy's story had touched her heart. Her brother was dealing with bladder cancer and I had been praying for him. God placed Harriet in my life and for that I felt blessed.

When Joy finally got to my house and read the letter for herself, she could do nothing but cry. She said it was as if a huge burden had been lifted from her shoulders and she then was made to realize God's purpose for her cancer. When her tears were controlled she said, "I can't explain how I feel except to say that I feel relief and peace as I have never felt before. If our story can help but one person to see beyond his circumstances to what is really important in life, then it will all be worthwhile. The cancer with all of its pain, cannot even make a dent in the joy I feel just now."

Joy was experiencing victory as never before and Satan had been buried. She was more alive than ever before even with the cancer that had ravaged her body. I knew then why I had written the book and I, too, felt a marvelous peace. To think that the same God who created the universe was allowing me to praise Him through this fashion, was more than I could have ever dreamed. *"But thanks be to God, who always leads us in triumphal procession in Christ and through us spreads everywhere the fragrance of the knowledge of Him"* (2 Corinthians 2:14).

In Him, we are victorious no matter what the circumstances, no matter what the disappointments. He was now entrusting us to spread His fragrance to others, despite our trials, through this book, and it was an awesome realization. We praised Him, and praised Him!

One by one, as the afternoon faded into the evening, I was able to complete my phone calls and share the good news. Everyone was thrilled and we rejoiced together in what the Lord had accomplished. Joy and I now had a new mission!

"Lord, thank you for giving me the opportunity of getting your Word out to people who don't know where to go in time of crisis. What a privilege to be your partner in this work through the book.

"Lord, if it took cancer in my life to let me be where I am today, then I praise you for allowing me to go through this time of fire, this battle.

"I have one more thing to say, Lord. *'It is well with my soul!!!'*"

Chapter 13

A New Church Family

In October of 1996, Jim and I joined the family of Faith Evangelical Presbyterian Church of Kingstowne, Virginia. After attending the church for almost five months, going through a new members' class and getting to know the congregation, we were convinced that this was God's plan for us. It had been a painful time in our lives and at times is still painful, but with each passing day I realize that this is exactly where God wants us to be.

Our church family is very loving, caring and supportive to Joy, my mother, and to our family. God knew I would need support to care for Joy and I had found it. Hardly a week goes by that someone doesn't call me and ask what they can do for me or for her. The family of God is just wonderful!

I joined the choir, along with Adam, Rita and Joy, and began singing again. Oh, the joy of music for me! I cannot tell you what it does for my soul. Only someone who loves music as much as I do can relate to what I feel. It is the biggest release for me when I sing. The music fills my soul and heart with praise. I thank God for the gift of music. Nothing else satisfies my heart in praise to Him quite like it. Our choir director asked me if I would consider directing for him at times when he is absent and I was thrilled. He is extremely talented and I consider it an honor to direct from time to time. The choir is filled with marvelous talent but along with their talent they are compassionate and kind and were very accepting of my directing limitations.

Singing in the choir with Joy, Adam and Rita is a marvelous blessing for me. Adam and I also sing together in the church praise band each Sunday morning and it is a cherished gift from God.

We sing great choruses of praise to Him and as I survey the congregation and see Joy singing with all that is within her despite her continuous battle, I am filled with love and worship for Jesus Christ. To stand next to my son and see how God has led in his life, I thank God once again. I am blessed.

Joy continued to take the chemotherapy, Navelbine, and still had her hair. For that, we were all very thankful. However, her blood counts were still low and she was getting Procrit injections three times a week. Her body was having a hard time producing enough red blood cells on its own and Procrit acts like the natural substance that your body needs to produce red blood cells. Just one more appointment to remember to make! Chemo was scheduled every Wednesday, Procrit on Mondays, Wednesdays and Fridays, and Arridia (the bone-strengthening treatment) once a month! Her condition remained status quo! She continued to sing praises to Him. *"Therefore ... stand firm. Let nothing move you. Always give yourselves fully to the work of the Lord, because you know that your labor in the Lord is not in vain"* (1 Corinthians 15:58).

I thank God for Faith Presbyterian Church. It is my lifeline! I needed the people and the support very much. I miss our friends at Grace but God knew it was time for me to move on and His timing was perfect. I will be ever grateful for the great truths of God's Word that I learned in my years at Grace and for the friendships I found there. "Thank you, Father."

Chapter 14

The Prize Arrives

While Christmas is always wonderful, Christmas of 1996 was not quite the same as in years past. Joy and I did virtually no shopping together because she was just too tired most of the time. She suffered from a cold that wouldn't quit and her cough was back. Due to my mother's continued recovery from her fall, I did all of her shopping as well as my own in snatches of time after work. Joy had to do the same thing with limited time. Nevertheless, the season was blessed as usual because the real meaning of Christmas has nothing to do with earthly gifts exchanged here on earth, but the marvelous gift of God's son free for the asking and accompanied by priceless treasures.

Joy's latest bone scan had revealed no new cancer in new places and the yearly and dreaded tests were over at least for a while. Her weight, though, continued to drop. I kept kidding her by telling her that she would soon be into my closet! She had gone from almost 200 pounds to 160! Foods just didn't appeal to her and the kind of food that did was just junk food, and she couldn't eat much of that. The chemotherapy dampens an appetite in a big way!

My additions and corrections to the manuscript had been noted and returned to the editors and we eagerly awaited the release of the book. That is all we talked about. Well, we did manage to discuss Adam and Rita's upcoming wedding (June 7) with great anticipation. Being the mother of the groom, especially at this time, definitely had its advantages although Joy and I were again making silk moiré roses for the wedding reception favors as we had done for Andrew and Julie's wedding. That project helped keep our minds occupied during the waiting process!

At long last I received a call from the editor at the publishing company saying my ten complimentary copies of the book had been shipped. The day arrived for UPS to deliver the package, but due to a mix up of some sort, it was delivered to another state! I was very disappointed! However, I had waited this long so a little longer would make no difference.

The very next day, I rushed home to find the package waiting at my front door. I didn't tell my mother that I was home because I wanted to be alone when I saw the book for the first time. I took the package and, like a child, quickly ran upstairs to my bedroom and shut the door. I don't know why but I sat with the package on my lap for the longest time. It was as though I couldn't quite believe what I had worked so hard for, and for so long, was finally becoming a reality. Maybe I was afraid that it would vanish if I opened it.

At long last I took a deep breath, prayed a hushed prayer, and opened it. It was beautiful! The cover was done in soothing yet vibrant shades of purple and teal. So simple and yet so majestic. It was my gift to Joy, my tribute to my family for their love and support during these critical years, and my testimony to my Lord and Savior Jesus Christ. How very humbled I felt. God was allowing me the honor of offering up my praise to Him through this beautiful book with the possibility of sharing it with many others. Well, it simply took my breath away! How I praised my glorious Lord!

Joy and Debby, a cousin of Jim's (Debby's husband Scott and Jim are cousins) and a true sister in the Lord, were both to come over to see the "prize." Debby had graciously offered to help with promotion of the book. She has been so supportive to us, not only in regards to the book but with Joy's physical needs as well. She is always there to meet any need that we might have and most importantly, she is a real prayer warrior. She and Scott and their sweet children, Gregory, Kelly and Tina, are very precious to our family as well as to Joy.

Scott made business cards for us and had written letters to various radio personalities to obtain interviews for us. He had shared the book with many people and had become a great spokesperson for us. Family is great!!

I ran downstairs just as the doorbell rang and there stood Debby with Gregory, Kelly and Tina all waiting to see "Aunt Sandy's book."

"Has Joy seen it yet?" Debby asked excitedly.

"Not yet," I replied, "but she is on her way."

"Maybe she should see it first before we do," Debby said, trying to hold back a bit on her enthusiasm much to the obvious displeasure of the three bright-eyed cherubs who were anxiously waiting to see it!

"Oh, no! She won't mind at all. She will be here very shortly, if she doesn't have an accident racing to get here!" I said with a laugh.

I presented the book to them and amidst "oohs" and "aahs," they, too, were clearly overwhelmed with the fruits of my labor. I felt so honored to have them share in my wonderful moment.

My mother was also looking at the "prize" and, although she said very little, I knew she was pleased for me. Mother, who through the years has found it difficult to put into words the things in her heart, told me later how very proud of me she was. It meant a lot to me.

How I would have liked for Mother to have been able to share in the joy of the book as she would have several years ago when she was in much better mental health. The depression had surfaced once again and she found it difficult to be joyous about anything at all. How my heart ached for her. I have come to realize that we are only responsible for our own happiness. We cannot be totally responsible for the happiness of another. We can add to their happiness, try to make them happy by acts of kindness, and so forth, and I have tried to do that over these last few years. You see, happiness depends on your circumstances but joy comes from the heart. We have to concentrate on the joy, true joy, that Christ gives us. The joy that comes from knowing Him and knowing that life here on this circle, beautiful as it is, is only temporary. Real joy is knowing that with Christ we have assurance of eternal life. Depression is Satan's way of clouding our thinking, thus robbing us of that joy. We must not let him do that. How I continually prayed that my mother would reach back for the joy that was buried so deeply within her.

The door flew open and in came Joy donning a baseball hat with the words "To Run The Race With Joy" emblazoned on the front. In her hands were hats for Debby, Scott, Jim and me. She placed hats on our heads and fairly shrieked, "Okay, where is it?"

As I placed it into her hands, she was clearly overcome with emotion. I knew her feelings, while different from mine in some ways, were in this instance so very much like mine. We were fighting this battle from two different perspectives, but we were fighting it together and because of that, we knew each other very well. We could almost anticipate each other's words and even thoughts so much of the time.

"Well," she said, with that twinkle in her eye, after spending time looking through the book, "I asked the Lord to let me live to see it published and now that it is finally here, I don't know what to say because I didn't ask anything beyond that!"

We laughed with her and assured her that God was not finished with her yet. We then rejoiced for some time and took lots of pictures. It was a wonderful time and a memory that will not be forgotten; the culmination of a dream for us all; the desire of my heart. *"Delight yourself in the Lord and He will give you the desires of your heart"* (Psalm 37:4).

Chapter 15

A New Ministry Begins

With the arrival of the book came the realization that we had a responsibility to market it. I knew nothing about marketing and neither did Joy or Debby. However, we were determined that we would learn all we could.

Joy, with her connections at NBC, began to do some research there for possibilities of exposure. Debby offered that area churches were a good place to start and she agreed to work on that aspect of marketing. Jim gave us ideas about contacting local Christian bookstores, some owners being clients of his, and he also graciously opened a business account for us under the name of SKR Promotions and placed seed money in it to help with expenses we were sure to incur. It was a new venture for us all and we were very excited.

The publisher called Debby and set up a conference call for us the next week to discuss the whole marketing concept and how they could help. We also contacted a local Christian bookstore and they were very excited as they offered to host a book-signing at their store. We scheduled it for Saturday, February 22. This was already beyond my wildest dreams and I was having a hard time comprehending the whole thing.

The next week at the prearranged time, I arrived at Debby's and we had our conference call with the publisher. He explained their plans for my book and then introduced us to our marketing coordinator in their office, Sherry Neuenschwander. It was their first attempt at hiring a marketing coordinator and I was her first assignment! Mr. Runk told me that we were to do everything through Sherry and that I would come to think of her as a sister. And that I have!

Sherry and I instantly "clicked." She had read my book, believed in the message I wanted to convey and felt a special bond with us even though we had not met face to face. I hung up from that meeting feeling great excitement for what was ahead. I wanted *To Run The Race With Joy* to touch people and give them hope through times of crisis, to let them see inside the workings of a family sold out to God and to let them witness the growth of those who are yielded to Him. And now we would begin to do just that.

Our first speaking engagement was held at Rose Hill Baptist Church before their Ladies Auxiliary. What a blessed group of women! We have come to think of them as a "family" because they have made us feel so welcome. At the conclusion of our presentation, we held our very first book-signing. What an exciting event! And the most important aspect of it was that many more women 'were now joining our prayer team. That was, by far, the most encouraging part of our new ministry — to realize that in every place we spoke, we were adding to our prayer team as well as offering hope and encouragement to many through our testimonies and the sharing of our story.

With the help of Sherry and locally with the help of Debby, Joy and I traveled from Florida to New York in one year with our ministry. We appeared on several radio and television shows and conducted numerous women's retreats. Joy's story touched many, many lives and her spirit has given hope to otherwise hopeless people. In the first year of publication, *To Run The Race With Joy* sold over 2,300 copies! Just when I begin to feel that perhaps this is all God wanted to do with the book, someone writes or calls us to tell us what the book has meant to them, people whom I've never met! I have just been amazed at the response.

Our first book-signing at a bookstore was very exciting. I remember covering my eyes as Jim drove past the bookstore to park the car and asking him: "Is anyone there?" I had this empty feeling that we would sit for two hours all alone with no one wanting to buy a book. Not that we haven't done that since the book has been published; that is to be expected when you are not a "known" author, but I just didn't want the first book-signing to be that way! To my surprise there were people waiting for us! And on that glorious February Saturday, we signed 65 books! After we left and in the next month, the store sold a total of 115 books.

Sherry arranged many book-signings and radio and television appearances for us. She worked very hard. What a great professional she is! And the most important thing, she is our sister in the Lord and prays for us continually. God has blessed our lives through knowing her. We wanted desperately to meet her; one of Joy's requests before God would choose to take her was to meet Sherry! God would honor her request but not for a year. In His time — in His time!

I love Sherry! and I haven't even met her yet. Sandy has talked with her on the telephone and we know God has chosen her especially for us. We are off on an exciting adventure and I am very excited. I had helped Sandy several years ago with our girls' group at Grace, and now we are to be a team once again. This is beyond wonderful.

I look forward to each new book-signing and speaking engagement with such joy. I prayed that God would send just the right people for us to minister to. Each time, He did! Even though we knew He would, we were always amazed. I have met so many wonderful people. And the great thing is that everywhere we went I left there knowing that there were that many more people praying for me. I will continue just as God wants me too. Praise His Name!!

Chapter 16

Reality Checks In Once Again

With all the excitement of the book being published and with our speaking engagements and book-signings, we had been able to shove Joy's cancer to the back of our minds, partly because she seemed to be doing so well and partly because it was easy to forget when she just refused to talk about anything negative and she had become such a master at disguising her pain. However, April 9, 1997 came and it was time for the dreaded bone scan!

The bone scan results were not good! Not good at all. It showed "extensive blastic matastases." More radiation was prescribed. As Joy read the results of the scan to me over the phone, all the pain and disappointment of previous times swept over my heart. My throat tightened as it always did and my mouth, as in times past, became painfully dry. What did I say to her? All my flippant quips of the past seemed inappropriate and my encouragement seemed empty and meaningless. I didn't feel encouraged or strong, only weak and full of pain.

"Well," she suddenly said, breaking the silence, "I am going to the hardware store to get some potting soil for our plants and I'll come by your school on my way to your house. We have to get those flowers planted today!"

Her spirits, even though a little dampened, were certainly not water-soaked as mine seemed to be! Life would go on and she would live it, again regardless of the news she had just received. Yes, she had cried when she called me. We had both cried! But she appropriated God's strength to herself and He had supplied it. "My grace is sufficient" had again prevailed in her life.

Joy breezed into my office a short time later and as we ate a quick lunch, she showed me the report and I reread what I had already known. I was hit afresh as to the magnitude of her disease and the extent to which it had spread.

"Maybe they could just put me in a capsule and radiate my whole body," she laughingly said. "That would seem to be the best thing. I mean, if they could just blast my whole body, for it seems that there are not too many places where cancer is not present."

"Oh," I interrupted, "I know of one place where it isn't present and I predict it never will be! Your jaw!"

After we wiped our eyes and our emotions were once again in check through the medicine of laughter, I asked her to honestly tell me what was on her mind. She lowered her eyes and softly said, "A wheelchair! I don't want to have to be in a wheelchair! That is the scariest thing for me."

I knew it was the fear of becoming dependent upon someone else for those things that she had always counted on doing for herself; her independence hung in the balance! But maybe God wanted that from her too — her independence. I already knew in my heart that if God wanted that, she would give it to Him, but it would not be without great inward pain.

We met at the mall later to get an ice cream cone and to focus on the present. She would continue with the same chemotherapy and begin her radiation and we would wait upon the Lord. Our new ministry would be strengthened through this latest turn of events. God would be glorified!

We bought shoes at the mall, she bought her ice cream cone and I cheated on my three day diet, vowing not to divulge that to Jim and Adam, my diet buddies. We laughed and giggled and were thrown back to a time when we only worried about things such as the perfect Christmas present, diets and clothes. We prayed for others who were going through times of crisis, about which we knew nothing, until now.

We arrived home and I started preparing dinner and went to finish a load of laundry. Life had to go on. It was funny that one could hear such devastating news only hours before, but dinner and laundry were a constant! Joy went outside to do some yard work, putting down top soil and planting her field flowers. The cooler than normal April air was perhaps what she needed to help her sort out her private thoughts, and a talk between her and her God was needed.

She was out of breath, as had become common for her, when she climbed up the stairs and found me putting the last of my clean laundry into the dresser drawers. She plopped down on my bed and we launched out on one of our long overdue girl talks. We just lay there for the longest time, each lost in her own thoughts. Then I spoke, breaking the silence.

"Did you ever, in a million years, think that we would be signing books and speaking to people all over the place about our friendship, our faith and your cancer and having people encouraged and their own faith strengthened by our story?"

"No," she said. "I never even dreamed it. But I just love it and I am sure this is my purpose for having cancer. I feel like I'm really helping people and glorifying God. I feel like the heavy burden of cancer has been lifted off my shoulders and it has become instead a mantle of service to God. That makes all the difference."

I was filled with pride as I realized just how far this girl had come in the six short years since she had first been diagnosed with her cancer. I spoke to her through tears.

"It isn't very often that a person gets to see someone that they have led to the Lord grow and mature in Him even in the face of death as you are. I'm very proud of you."

"That means a lot to me," she said, with silvery tears cascading down her cheeks.

We were soon laughing and talking about how we would get on the *Oprah Show* to discuss our book. It was to be her ultimate goal, to reach as many people as we possibly could in the time God had left for her.

"I'll wear a dress," she volunteered, "if we get on television."

"A dress would be nice," I retorted, knowing full well it would be a sacrifice because she loves her jeans! "Very nice."

We went downstairs, found my mother awake from her usual afternoon nap, and talked with her as we completed dinner preparations. We would discuss Joy's test results at dinner, but with our renewed spirits it would be easier.

Jim offered his usual upbeat thoughts and encouragement at the news but later when we were alone, we confided to each other our concerns that her time here might not be long. We had been negotiating for several months on a house at the beach and we knew if that came into being it would push our focus into another direction and Joy would love being a part of that. It would give her something to look forward to. Jim was a firm believer in goals and focus — something to anticipate. Our new ministry through my book was our spiritual focus and the beach property would be our recreational focus. It would be good!

My mother, because of her depression, could not find a focus. Hard as we tried, we could not help her to find one. It was still at the center of my heart — her depression. I continued to pray daily for wisdom. She did seem to sparkle a bit when we discussed Adam and Rita's upcoming wedding, but unfortunately the sparkle never lasted too long. I took her shopping for a new dress for the wedding and we had a wonderful time. For a while she did forget about her sadness. How I prayed to have my mother back! Why couldn't I understand this thing called "depression" that was daily claiming the joy of so many? My mother spent so much time concentrating on dying that she couldn't enjoy living! I thanked God for each happy time that we shared; however, I still felt as though I had failed miserably every time she slipped back into the sadness even though I knew in my heart that I wasn't responsible. The role reversal of mother-daughter was very bitter for me but a role that most of us will one day have to play — like it or not! I still would not have her live anywhere else and I still thanked God for the privilege of caring for her, that was for sure!

Sherry had set up an engagement for us in my hometown of Charleston, West Virginia. We were to be present at the grand opening of a Family Christian Bookstore for a book-signing and we were to speak in my home church and do a local television spot. I had talked my mother and Adam into going with us as well as my sister. Mother was getting excited at visiting with her sisters and Joy was feeling pretty good. It was to be our first "road trip."

The book-signing was great and very exciting. My cousins and my aunt and uncle came to the mall to see us and we sold and signed lots of books. We had a marvelous trip. It was special because my mother was able to share in the experience with me. I knew she was proud of me!

Joy did very well on the trip except for the constant pain in her back. That did worry us all. We took advantage of the whirlpool provided at the motel where we stayed, but it was of little help. Radiation would begin when we returned to Virginia.

I praised God for yet another opportunity for witness, and for the strength He had given to Joy; however, I also prayed for the added strength I knew we would all need once we were back home.

The results of my bone scan are not good. Cancer is in my back, big time! No wonder I have been in so much pain! My back hurts almost all the time. I'm scared! I don't want a wheelchair. "Please, Lord, not a wheelchair." Sandy and I talked it out and shared our feelings. I will miss her, Lord!

We had a great time in West Virginia. I love Sandy's relatives. It was nice to have Nina, Adam and Carolyn with us. The trip was nice but my back hurt so bad. I didn't want to say how much. God will carry me.

Chapter 17

Our Availability

Today, April 22, 1997, I am very discouraged! Our first trip was very successful and most encouraging for us all, but our impending visit to Joy's doctor tomorrow made me realize that the focus of our ministry dealt with Joy's cancer. It was real and the time had come to face it again.

I called my cousin Debby just to talk. It was so wonderful to have a sister in the Lord who was so available and so easy to talk to. As I poured my heart out to her, she listened and comforted me with words that only God could have given to her — and just for me. I told her of my discouragement and fear of the news our appointment might bring. I know we are not supposed to worry about tomorrow for tomorrow will take care of itself — so difficult to do — so very difficult. The "fixer" in me had surfaced once again and I cannot fix this! I felt so tired, so vulnerable. I kept thinking, I can't do this, I just can't do this anymore! I knew I had to draw upon the strength of the Lord as never before. I just had to be available. He would sustain me.

Debby offered to go with us to the appointment and I gratefully accepted her offer. I thanked God for Debby and for her sensitivity to my heart. It would be good to have someone else with me to help bear this sometimes unbearable situation. I felt so very weak at this time. My devotion for the day came racing back to my memory. It was taken from Exodus 4. Moses doubted his ability and he concentrated on his weaknesses, but God said unto him, *"Who gave man his mouth? Who gives him sight or makes him blind? Is it not I, the Lord? Now go; I will help you speak and will teach you what to say."* As God met the need of Moses, He would meet my needs and send help to me as I needed it. Truly, Debby was one whom the Lord sent to me and I would forever praise Him for that gift. She would never realize the burden that she had lifted from my very heavy heart with just that one phone conversation. The "household of faith" is a treasure from God!

I finished up at the high school and walked to my car in weather too cool and gray to be April. It seemed a perfect setting for my still slightly dampened spirit.

After dinner, Jim and I went outside to do a little much needed yard work. The sun had broken through the clouds for a while and I needed to be outside in the cool air. I pulled weeds in Joy's tulip garden and in the rose garden we had planted together. The tulips were vibrant in color and yet so fragile. The rose bushes were alive with new growth and promises of beautiful blooms in the next few weeks. We had planted a rose bush in honor of each family member. Mom's was, of course, delicate pink, mine was luscious coral, Andrew and Julie had a velvety red one; Jim's was regal white. For Adam (and soon Rita), we chose a deep rich pink. For Joy, last but not least, the color was a sunny bright yellow, her favorite color! We had had so much fun picking the colors for everyone.

Working with the roses, my mind flashed back to a day which now seemed so far away when, as we were planting them, Joy looked up and said to me, "When I'm gone, remember how much fun we had planting and watching our beautiful roses grow. I think God will let me see them from time to time, so take care of them and each year when they bloom and you are out here tending to them, remember that I'll be here too!"

A lonely feeling washed over my soul as I recounted that day and I realized that the time may be nearing when the Lord would call her home. But somehow amidst the loneliness, I felt peace working in the garden — our garden. We will face tomorrow hard as it might be. With God we would not be alone — never would we be alone. His promises are sure. He just wants our availability.

92

God says, *"I am with you always"* (Matthew 28:20). Isn't it great that there is One who never changes and who is always with us? He is my fortress and my Rock in the raging waves on the sea of life. *"Build your hopes on the Rock that will stand secure in high winds, heavy rains and roaring floods"* (Matthew 7:24). "Help me, Lord, to hold your hand and not be afraid of what may lie ahead for me." I will trust Him who will go with me through the black and surging currents of death's stream.

"I am with you always" is enough for my soul to live on!

Chapter 18

Let Your Light So Shine

April 23, 1997, and the day had arrived for us to go to the doctor to get whatever news we must. Once again while in the waiting room, we laughed and talked and nobody would have known the heaviness of our hearts. Joy truly seemed oblivious to it all.

Dr. Peter West, her radiologist, met with us. He was so gentle and it was very apparent that he had such great admiration for Joy. She never failed to give God the glory for even so-called "bad news." So when he told her that her cancer in her back was much too advanced for standard radiation, nothing changed for Joy. She just said, "So what now?"

He told us about a treatment, an injection, called Strontium 89 Metastron which had shown promising results. The cost per injection — $2,500!!! WOW, some injection!! He did advise it for Joy and was confident her insurance company would at least pay for part of it. It was the only choice she had. Dr. West would administer the injection himself. Joy said, "Let's do it!"

Debby was amazed at the respect and love shown to Joy on that visit. She hadn't gone to an appointment with us before and even though I had told her, she said she never imagined that Joy's testimony had been so powerful. We praised God but we shed a lot of tears together for what would lie ahead for Joy.

God's Word tells us in Matthew 5:16 *"... let your light shine before men that they may see your good works and praise your Father in heaven."* Joy's "light" was her cancer, of all things. Never before could I have imagined cancer as that "light." It was the brightest "light" I had ever seen. It would be a long time before I could see the rainbow reflected by that "light" through the tears that streamed down my face that day.

Chapter 19

A Flesh And Blood Answer

Before we left the doctor's office, I had asked one of Joy's oncology nurses, who I knew would tell me the truth straight up, to give me the bottom line! She told me that things were very bleak for Joy. She could live perhaps another year, but she was deteriorating and she could only get worse, barring a miracle. There was also the possibility that I would be giving her growth factor injections once again. All of this was only prolonging the inevitable.

I felt myself once more crashing emotionally but the ministry God had just entrusted to us had to be continued for however long God wanted. I couldn't let anything get in the way of that. God would provide the strength I needed just as surely as He would provide the strength Joy needed.

Joy and I went to choir practice that evening but I didn't feel much like singing. Even when Joy made her silly noises and funny remarks which we did with great regularity, my heart wasn't in it. Quickly realizing my deflated spirit, she punched me in the side and whispered, "Come on, girlfriend, give it up! We will get through this. Let's sing!"

It was hard not to smile when she was around but, try as I might, I really couldn't put my heart and soul into the music that night! The events of the day played over and over in my head. I was glad when practice was over and I could go home.

God's timing is always so perfect. Very soon after that night, Teri, Joy's cousin whom she grew up with and thought of as a sister, called me one day to discuss Joy's prognosis. We had been talking on a regular basis concerning Joy, but this time she wanted to talk about becoming involved in a much more significant way.

97

Teri told me she had been moved and touched by the book. "I could have been there, but I wasn't," she tearfully said. "We weren't there. None of us was there. I know we all have our own lives and things are hectic, but we could have helped, we could have pushed. She is our family. Maybe we didn't realize how sick she really is, but now that I see through her story how it has been for her and for you and your family, I want to be there for her and for you, too, if you want me!"

I felt as though a weight had been lifted from around my neck. God's answer for strength came in a flesh and blood form. I didn't expect it. How precious to have someone else to share the responsibility — her family. I praised God for such a marvelous answer to prayer. I couldn't wait to call Debby to share the news with her. We would have additional help — a link with her family. We praised God together for His answer.

Joy was thrilled to have Teri back in her life with the promise of such a commitment. We asked Teri if she also wanted to be a part of our ministry team and she was very happy that we had asked. We were all so excited about our "team" that it was as though we had forgotten what gave us the privilege of doing this — cancer! Our light was now Joy's light and even though we didn't like it, God had chosen it for us, for now. His ways are not our ways.

For my thoughts are not your thoughts, neither are your ways my ways, declares the Lord. As the heavens are higher than the earth, so are my ways higher than your ways and my thoughts than your thoughts. As the rain and the snow come down from heaven, and do not return to it without watering the earth and making it bud and flourish, so that it yields seed for the sower and bread for the eater, so is my word that goes out from my mouth: It will not return to me empty, but will accomplish what I desire and achieve the purpose for which I sent it. You will go out in joy and be led forth in peace; the mountains and hills will burst into song before you, and all the trees of the field will clap their hands. Instead of the thorn bush will grow the pine tree, and instead of briers the myrtle will grow. This will be for the Lord's renown, for an everlasting sign, which will not be destroyed. — Isaiah 55:8-13

I love Teri with all my heart. She is the only biological family I have left because of circumstances that I choose not to discuss. I feel like she is my sister. We grew up closer than sisters and then, because sometimes your lives go in different directions, we lost that closeness we once had. I have missed it, especially now since my mom's death, I feel a need for my family. Sandy and Jim have been family, don't get me wrong. I love them like they are family. But I mean someone who I grew up with and knows me like Teri does. Do you understand? Anyhow I am very happy that she will be helping Sandy and Debby and everyone with my care.

I love Teri and Kevin's children, Tiffany, Trisha and especially my little guy, Tyler. People say he looks like me! I don't know if that is true but I like hearing it. I wish I could live to see him grow up. I gave him a copy of my book and signed it. My dearest wish for him is to accept the Lord as his Savior and to live for Jesus.

I pray for Teri and her family every day and my desire is that they know and love the Lord so they can spend eternity with me. It won't be long until the Lord takes me home, but until then I'll keep praying.

I'm so happy that Teri will also be helping with the book. She will be going with us on our retreats and when we talk about the book to women's groups. "Thank you, Lord, for letting my ministry include Teri — it means so much to me!"

Chapter 20

Beaches

Jim and I had for some time been looking for a rental property to purchase when we sold Jim's home place. We have for years been spending our summers in Bethany Beach, Delaware, with our sons, their families and, of course, Joy. Therefore the obvious choice for our family was Bethany Beach. Everyone was excited at the prospect of having our own beach place. Not just to have for a week each summer, but to be able to spend more family time there all during the year. So when the home place sold, Jim and I headed for Delaware and the community where we had always rented.

The rest of our family were not prepared for the property we decided to purchase there! It looked like a disaster — a real "fixer-uper" if there ever was one! But Jim, who can see things as they "can be" instead of the way they are, and I, who fell in love with the location (right on the water) and the fact that there would be lots and lots of room for us all, felt this was just perfect for us! It would require a lot of hard work, but we had done it before and we could do it again.

We had been renting a summer home in the same community where we had just bought for about six years. We always had said if we ever had the opportunity to buy our own home we would like for it to be on the water across the pond from where we rented. This had to be from God, for when indeed that opportunity presented itself, the only property available in that wonderful community was a house "across the pond." A challenge though it was, it was meant for us and never was I more sure of that.

Joy went with us to the settlement. The minute she saw our house, she fell in love with it, work and all. As we stood on the dock, she and I looked across the water which was glistening like a sea of diamonds in the bright sunlight. As she gazed up at the bright azure blue sky she broke our silence and said, "I could die here. I really could."

It was on Memorial Day, 1997, that we settled on our "challenge." Joy and I spent three weeks there after school was out for the summer. Jim and the boys did a lot of work on weekends and Jim drove back and forth during the week so he could, as he put it, "Keep my practice going so I can continue to make money for you all to spend and, of course, to be able to eat!"

At the end of those three weeks we were all exhausted, especially Joy. However, she enjoyed every moment of our time there. Even though I knew she was in agony much of the time, you would never have known it looking at her. We painted, cleared the yard, front and back, of fifty bags of trash (yes fifty!!). We painted and planted flowers. Oh, did I mention that we painted, and painted and painted some more? The entire house inside and out had to be painted. We hired the painting to be done on the outside, but all of us together painted the inside. I have pictures of Joy lying on the bed and, using an extension handle for the roller, painting a wall. Nothing stopped her. We shopped for dressers, beds and furniture at local stores and flea markets. It was looking good! Even we were amazed at how much difference we could make with just a little paint — well, a lot of paint — and elbow grease — lots and lots of elbow grease.

The kids were getting more and more excited every time we made an improvement. It soon became apparent to them also that this was a great idea — crazy, but great!

Neighbors would drive by and commend us on how great a job we were doing. And speaking of neighbors, we were blessed to have neighbors who were Christians. Gerrie and Vince Ciecielski were our next door neighbors. How much we loved them right from the very start. Gerrie had been praying for Christian neighbors and was thrilled when God answered her prayers. We became instant friends and to this day we remain so. She fell in love with

Joy and our book and has shared it with many of her friends. God is so very good.

During those three weeks, Jim would spend two or three days at a time back in Virginia in his law practice, but Joy and I stayed in Bethany because we wanted to continue to work on the house. We spoke to him daily and gave him reports on our progress. He cautioned us all the time to pace ourselves but we usually worked until very late at night and were up very early every morning to get started on the day's activities. We were just too pumped to pace ourselves. We played our "oldies" on the radio and laughed, worked and talked. We only went out to eat a couple of times. Most of the time we just fixed quick meals and worked!

One night we were just too tired to work after dark and so we put on the movie *Beaches* and laughed and cried together as we had done many times before while watching it. This time it was too real. We cried even harder realizing that her time was probably close. The difference in us and the movie was Jesus Christ. We know we will see each other again. Joy's death will not be final! It will only be a separation. How sad when I think that without Jesus Christ, people have no hope — all the pain and no hope! She asked me if she had to go to a Hospice facility, would I be with her. I promised her that I would. Her fear was being in her last days without loved ones around. "You know that we will all be there!" I assured her. "We will always be there." She smiled and wiped away a tear that ran down her cheek. I dried up my own tears and we went to bed.

As I tumbled into bed and thought about the conversation we had just shared, I wondered what her thoughts were that night while alone with her God. I know she prays for healing as we all do. She has accepted God's will for her life, but how she does love life!

I turned off my light and slipped down into my pillow. I reached out and touched Jim's pillow and longed for our "snuggle time" together. I missed him but maybe I needed to spend this time with Joy. She seemed to need to talk a lot and we were doing much of that as only girls can. I thanked my Lord for this place and for my husband and our family, and for my friend who in the next room was perhaps crying out to God and coming to terms once again with the frailty of life and its preciousness. *"Take my life and let it be consecrated, Lord, to thee"* (Frances Ridley Havergal).

"I pray to be healed of my cancer, Lord. I don't mean to be selfish. It is my heart's desire.

"One day at a time! You hold tomorrow in your hands. I have no guarantees. Lord, I want to be healed so badly. I don't know what you have for me up ahead as each day unfolds. But my heart is ready for whatever you have for me because I can hold your hand and you are holding mine.

"I'm so very tired, Lord. I hurt so much. I want to be normal again! But, your will Lord. Your will be done!"

Chapter 21

The Wedding

There was much excitement over the beach house, but the real excitement was Adam and Rita's wedding. We settled on our house Memorial Day; "our" wedding was to be June 7.

We spent weeks preparing for the wedding and eagerly looked forward to a new daughter in our family. Rita comes from a large family — three brothers, a sister, and many nieces and nephews. They were all crazy about Adam and he, them.

Adam and Rita had decided to get married up in Northern Virginia where we live rather than down close to Richmond where she came from. Her family was in total agreement and so we proceeded with the plans. I tried to help Rita's mom as much as I could because I knew it was hard to plan a wedding when you live over two hours from where it would take place. Bettie (Rita's mother) and I talked lots on the phone and she asked me to help her decide on a place for the reception. We had fun together planning a "perfect" wedding.

Bettie loved Joy and included her in the plans as well. Joy wanted to buy the wedding cake, and help Rita pick out bridesmaids' dresses. She was excited to be a part of it and, since Rita lived with her, she had come to think of Rita as a little sister. I knew Joy would miss Rita when she moved. I also could see that this event was helping Joy to stay "normal" as she so much wanted to do. God's timing — again so perfect.

The wedding day was cooler than normal for June but nothing could dampen our spirits. Rita was gorgeous and Adam was obviously ready for the event! He fairly beamed when he saw her for the first time coming down the aisle. Tears were evident in his eyes.

Andrew, who had walked me down the aisle earlier, served as best man and he, too, had tears in his eyes as he stood beside his brother. Julie looked absolutely beautiful as she joined the wedding party. I was so proud of the four of them. They are such good friends and now "family" — our family. Mother was lovely and very happy to have lived to see her "baby" grandchild married. She had been a very special part of his life and he had been special to her. I thanked God for my mother's part in our sons' lives. They are the young men they are today in large part because of her influence.

As Rita and Adam led the recessional, they kissed us and handed letters accompanied by white rose buds, to us and to Rita's parents. Completely unexpected, Adam returned to the front to escort me from the church. What a beautiful symbol of respect for me as his mother. I was touched beyond words. I cannot share with you the contents of those priceless letters except to say that as Andrew had let us know by our precious conversations with him just before his wedding how much our family meant to him. Adam, too, was letting us know that he cherished his childhood and our family and wanted those same values for his family as well. How very proud we were of our sons. "Thank you, Father, for the blessings of our children."

My heart overflowed with praises that day — ceaseless praises to Jesus Christ. *"... Is anyone happy? Let him sing songs of praise"* (James 5:13b).

I was tired but so happy today for Adam and Rita. It was a beautiful wedding. Chip and I had a good time.

"Thank you Lord for Chip's friendship and for the friendship of his family, too. Lord bless Adam and Rita as they serve you together and thank you especially for allowing me to be there today. I love you, Lord."

Chapter 22

God's Strength Personalized

It was during this time that one of my dearest friends, Mary, entered into a serious depression. I felt so sorry for her. We have been friends since 1987. She is a school health aide as I am, but she works in an elementary school. We had been having some pretty in-depth discussions for some time and I had been praying for her but I could tell that her problems were going way beyond what I could help her solve.

My mother, with her depression, had seemed some better. I talked to her about Mary and of course she understood completely. I suggested medical help to Mary but she still felt that she could overcome it. The breakup of her marriage of some forty years and the prospect of being on her own for the first time in a long time, was more than she could endure. I could only pray. I wanted to become more involved but I realized with my mother and Joy, I could only give so much. I felt completely helpless and as time went by I realized that I had to take matters into my own hands and get help for Mary.

I decided to call Mary's sister (someone whom I had never met) in North Carolina and tell her of my fears for Mary. She was so grateful that I had called because she didn't realize that things were so bad. Mary hadn't wanted to worry her and therefore had not told Nikki the real truth about her depression. With encouragement from Nikki, Mary took a leave of absence from work and went to North Carolina to stay with her sister and brother-in-law for a while. It was the best thing she could have done. I couldn't be there for Mary the way she needed, and God's answer was Mary's sister. I thanked God for Nikki and her husband and the wonderful way in which they cared for my friend. I thanked God for giving me the wisdom to be able to admit that I couldn't do for Mary what she needed. Nikki got professional help and medicine for Mary and today she has been healed. Back at work and church, she is closer to the Lord than ever before and she gives God the glory. She is strong and healthy and much wiser. Her divorce is now final, but God is helping her to realize that if she depends on Him, she is never alone. I am so proud of her. She has been a great support to me with my mother and with Joy. She is a constant and wonderful friend. It's good to have her back.

Praise God for the lessons I'm learning in knowing when to ask for help and when to "allow" God to use someone else because He really doesn't need me to do it all. To borrow a phrase I heard someone once say, "Lord, I am now resigning as general manager of the universe." That sounds like the words of someone just like me. "Lord, may I truly 'resign' and not take my resignation papers back!"

During this time, Joy was enjoying freedom from pain in her back as a result of that very expensive injection. We were very grateful for a little reprieve from that pain. Of course, chemotherapy continued. We were concerned because Joy's blood counts continued to drop and she needed platelets more and more frequently. She called that an "oil change." Also her left knee became excruciatingly painful. She decided she would tell the doctor about her knee at our next visit because I told her I would tell him if she didn't!

Debby and I took her to the doctor for that October 23 visit. The news was not good. She had seven new lesions on her left knee and, most likely, cancer was elsewhere in her body. She would need a new chemotherapy. Her doctor named off all the chemo therapies she had already had and the list seemed endless. I looked at Debby and her face said it all — what was left? The doctor couldn't tell us at that time what the new treatment would be. He said he would take her chart home and think about it over the weekend as to what the next step would be. He did order radiation on her left knee.

As with each visit, Debby and I questioned the doctor as to the wisdom of Joy's living by herself, driving, etc., and each time the answer was the same: "Joy is capable of deciding whether or not she can walk the stairs in her place or not, and she can certainly do what she feels like doing."

Of course Joy gave us that smirky "I told you so" look as she always did when she got her way. It was exactly what we had expected this time — the doctor's answer was the same, with the exception of his admonition concerning her driving. He advised her not to drive any more than was absolutely necessary and to consider very carefully whether or not she felt it safe to drive with so much pain in her left knee. She assured him she would know when she should stop driving. I knew that would be the last vestige of her independence to go; it would surely be by far the most difficult decision she had to make! We would just pray for wisdom!

As we sat in the waiting room for Joy to make her next doctor's appointment, a patient asked us if we were with the "famous Joy" and if she was always so cheerful and upbeat. When we replied that she was, the patient said, "I have been here often and have seen Joy countless times. I have never seen her cry or sad. She just doesn't seem to ever be down. She is an inspiration to us all!"

Debby and I smiled and agreed that Joy was a special person. We wiped away our tears and tried to get "it" back together again so that we didn't discourage Joy. We agreed there and then that she was indeed the "famous Joy."

The doctor had also told Joy that with the new chemotherapy he would choose, she would most likely lose her hair again. She had had hair for two years and now she would lose it again! "Well," she said, "I had hair all summer long so it won't be too bad." Debby and I decided we would buy coonskin caps when I went to Luray again, and when she lost her hair, the three of us would wear them together. Joy liked that idea.

We left the office that day with the "famous Joy" and laughed all the way home about our coonskin caps and our other great ideas for Joy's about-to-be-again-bald head. Laughter had become the best medicine of all for the three of us.

111

The strength that God had given to both of my dear friends, Mary and Joy, was of different kinds but exactly right for each of them. The strength he gives to Debby and to me is of an even different variety and yet He gives and gives until we are strong even when we are at our weakest. The kind of strength He gives to us is equipped and fashioned for us individually and is drawn from His inexhaustible reserves. How Great Thou Art!

Chapter 23

Independence Wanes

It became apparent when Joy and I went to Florida for a road trip the end of October, 1997, that Joy would very soon need help to walk. She couldn't even walk from our hotel across the street to the closest restaurant. I had to practically carry her! She was in constant pain.

These trips were always mingled with excitement as well as with fear. I always wondered what I would do if she really got sick and we were so far away from her doctor. I knew that God would provide if that happened, but I was always glad to get back home.

On Thursday night before our television interview, Joy was in terrible pain. Her left knee was much worse. I knelt beside her bed and prayed fervently for her. I prayed for a good night's sleep for her and a lessening of the pain. She was crying and I was crying for her. It was one of her lowest points! She took her medicine and we turned off the light. I continued to pray silently for her and soon her cries subsided and she drifted off to sleep.

The next morning she awoke and looked very well rested. I realized that I hadn't heard her up during the night. She said she slept like a baby for the first time in a while and the pain was much much better! We prayed together and thanked God for such a marvelous answer to prayer.

Our interview went smoothly. We were guests on the *Herman and Sharron Bailey Show.* They were so wonderful to us and we were privileged to be able to share our story with their vast audience and to promote our book.

Later, after the broadcast, we had lunch with my oldest brother, David, and his wife who live in Plant City, Florida. They drove to

113

Clearwater to meet us. David always makes Joy laugh. After lunch they left for home and we drove to the beach and did some sightseeing. It had been a very exciting time for us but Joy was exhausted when we finally fell into bed that evening after thanking God for providing her with a relatively pain-free knee for the day!

I praised God for His strength as we landed safely back at the airport in Washington, D.C., two days later, and for Jim as he met us to take us home. Being away from him was the most difficult thing for me. We are usually inseparable and I like it that way! I was so grateful for his support and encouragement to us in this ministry. We chattered all the way home about our trip and experiences and we giggled as we told him it would have been much more fun with him. I don't think he believed us at all!!

Once home in Virginia, Joy was to begin yet another chemotherapy carefully chosen by Dr. Beveridge called Novantrone. Her first treatment was to be November 12, and unexpected news — she might only have thinning hair this time — news she received with great joy! Radiation on her knee was scheduled for November 6.

She came by my office on her way home after being marked for her radiation and ate lunch with my nurse, Harriet, and me. Harriet suggested to her that she might benefit from a cane to help her weakened left knee. I wondered how she would take that suggestion, but to my surprise, she seemed to like it, especially after she confessed to us that she had fallen in the radiologist's office earlier that day (a fact she was going to avoid telling me). She agreed to get a cane that very afternoon.

During lunch, she recounted to Harriet and me the process of being marked for radiation. No butterflies or roses, only dots and very painful ones at that. She had secretly confided to me once that she had always wanted a tattoo but after her experience with being marked for radiation, all desires for one disappeared. She was completely cured. "It's painful!" she announced to us. "Very painful! Why anyone would want to do that and not have to, is crazy to me." Of course, Harriet and I had encountered lots of that "craziness" working in the high school!

Isn't it like sin, I thought. We sometimes have to feel the pain of it in order to want to avoid it. You can warn people of sin's effect on them but sometimes they just have to dabble in it for themselves and feel the pain before they are convinced. Often, we know sin can lead to consequences far beyond our pain. But even with that knowledge, it doesn't seem to deter some people from wanting to try it for themselves. Our free will is a wonderful thing — a wonderful gift from God — but we must stay close to Him to exercise it properly and to use it for our own good. It makes me realize how we need to keep in daily constant contact with the Father. Some of our frustration and exhaustion may be the result of the detours we take off the path God has placed us on. *"Blessed is the man who does not walk in the counsel of the wicked or sit in the seat of mockers. But his delight is in the law of the Lord, and on his law he meditates day and night"* (Psalm 1:1, 2).

Paul tells us in Hebrews 12:2 that Jesus Christ is the *"Author and finisher of our faith."* He must be our top priority. Our pain helps us to grow but sometimes it blinds us and leads us so far off the track that we are not following the right goal. We must pray through our pain and learn from it as did Job. We must run our race with authority.

115

I am so disappointed about the new lesions found on my left leg because I am afraid I will soon not be able to walk. My greatest fear is a wheelchair! "Lord, please do not make me that dependent. I fell today in my kitchen and I had a hard time getting up. I just fell! I just sat there in the middle of the floor and cried. I also fell in the doctor's office. Why Lord? Why, must I lose my legs? I cried for the longest time.

"Sandy and I are going to Florida to do a television program and to promote the book. I need to be strong, Lord! I am so tired. I know you will provide, Lord. You always do. Help us to do our best in Florida. I am excited. I pray for Sandy because I know she is scared every time we go away from home because she feels responsible. I know you know that too, Lord. Help me not to miss any opportunity to share what you have done for me. Take away my fear!"

Chapter 24

Back To College

The trips continued, one after another. God's strength was evident! Sherry had set up a trip for Joy and me to Nashville, Tennessee, for Joy to speak at her alma mater, Trevecca Nazarene University. Joy was so excited.

"When I think of all the times when I was in college that I tried to get out of going to chapel and now I am speaking there!" she said impishly, when she found out we were going. "It makes me feel so proud. I can show you all around Nashville and where I spent my college days."

We were scheduled to stay at the alumni house. We flew out of National Airport November 15, and were to catch a connecting flight out of Chicago. However, due to snow in Chicago, we were diverted to Cincinnati. Consequently, we didn't arrive at Trevecca until almost midnight!

Surprisingly, Joy did really well and wasn't too tired. We had reserved a wheelchair at the airports and at the university for her and she willingly used it. We could never have made it without the wheelchair! I thought she would really fight it but her desire to participate in our ministry was far greater than her fear of the wheelchair. I praised God for her change of heart because it was very apparent that we were going to go nowhere without the wheelchair — at least not far and certainly not in a timely fashion.

I wheeled her all over Nashville and took great glee going down hills and letting the chair go — ever so briefly — for a roller coaster effect! She told me I had far too much power, but we laughed hysterically every time I did it. We visited the Opryland Hotel. We could never have made it through even a quarter of the lobby had we not used the wheelchair! What fun we had! We encountered many strange looks as I performed my shenanigans with the wheelchair! Tired as Joy was at the end of the day, we made the most of our short sightseeing trip.

The next day we met with Jan Greathouse, our contact at the university. What a wonderful time we had with her. She had read our book and had written an article in their magazine *The Treveccan*, which featured Joy and Willard Scott on the front cover. She was excited to meet us finally and she and her husband treated us royally. Joy spoke at the university chapel before the student body. We had lunch with the president of the university and then did a book-signing at the university bookstore where we sold a number of books and signed them for the students. The next evening we spoke at Jan's women's Bible study and on Sunday evening we addressed the largest Nazarene church in Nashville. It was a wonderful trip and most memorable for both of us.

We left Nashville with memories that would last forever. We knew there were many more people praying for Joy. Jan would always be in our hearts — it was sad to leave her, but it was wonderful to know we would spend eternity with her some day!

Another trip had come to an end and again God had provided strength for Joy — strength that could have come no other way. It seemed with each trip Joy became stronger and more confident in her spirit. She was more determined than ever to use every opportunity we were given to go wherever God led us and for however long He chose, to praise Him through her cancer. Our ministry was clearly God's will for our lives. We were living Isaiah 49:31:

But those who hope in the Lord will renew their strength. They will soar on wings like eagles; they will run and not grow weary, they will walk and not be faint.

Chapter 25

Roses In December

Our annual Thanksgiving at our cabin in Luray was great, as usual. My sister Carolyn and her husband Mark came. I realized that without their girls and their families there to share it with us as in years before, it was hard for Carolyn. But the boys were there with their families (Rita's first as our "daughter"), and of course Mother and Joy were there. Our Thanksgiving Day together was blessed and Mother and Joy seemed to be almost normal. We had much to be grateful for!

One of our former pastors, W. Carl Miller, and his wife Betty, both whom we love dearly, always visited us in Luray during the Thanksgiving weekend. Their daughter Linda lives near Luray and they visit her each year. This year was no exception. They came to our house the Friday after Thanksgiving. We look forward to our reunions and it's always as if we had never been apart! The family of God is really awesome!

This year, however, Joy spent their entire visit upstairs in bed. She was just too tired to enjoy company. They had been praying for her for some time and I knew they understood her absence and would continue to pray. The rest of us, including my mother, who considered them her "kids" too, had a great visit with them. Some time ago, I purchased a magnet from a gift shop with the words, "God gives us memories so we will have roses in December." I keep it on my kitchen window sill. I was gathering some roses for coming Decembers with their visit.

With Thanksgiving over, Christmas was nearing, but I just couldn't get into the spirit at all. The thought of shopping seemed so overwhelming. Joy couldn't go at all and my mother really didn't seem to want to go.

During Pastor Smith's (Dr. Graham Smith retired and Pastor Neil Smith, no relation, was now our pastor) sermon the first Sunday in December, he asked us to reflect on the true meaning of Christmas ... "forgive us our Christmases as we forgive those who Christmas against us." It made me feel ashamed that I had let things like decorating and baking and Christmas shopping, and all the hoopla, overshadow my Savior's birthday! I determined in my heart that Sunday to change my attitude — to make it a special Christmas for everyone despite the circumstances. The truth of Christmas had never changed!

Jim had stayed home from church on that Sunday, December 7, to take Joy to get platelets because her blood counts were dangerously low. The day before, she had slept at our house almost all day despite her efforts to stay awake while I made her favorite cookies. She fought it when she was scheduled to have the platelets on a Sunday but she was just too weak to put up much of a fight.

My mother continued to be more confused and frail. But despite that, how could I ever have imagined that this would be the last Christmas I would have her! Nothing could have prepared me for that. What would I have done differently had I known? So many things — so very many things. I would never know until five months later just how glad I was that I had convinced her to go shopping with me one day in early December nor how glad I would be that I had heard and applied to my life that sermon Pastor Neil had preached to my heart.

I took a couple of hours off work and picked her up that day for the promised shopping trip. I took her to the mall and wheeled her all around each level to let her see the beautiful decorations. We laughed, shopped and had a great time. I made several trips to the car to take our purchases. As we laughed each time I loaded a mountain of packages on her lap and wheeled her to the car, she seemed like herself — for a while. We ate dinner together and talked and talked about everything and nothing. I didn't realize then how I would cherish that blessed afternoon. Joy had asked to go along (how I would have managed that, will remain a mystery!), but I was really glad that I had insisted I had to go with Mom — just she and I!

I had allowed myself time to cry several weeks previously as I mourned the Christmases past with Mom and Joy the way it used to be. But that afternoon made me so glad for the times we had left. I didn't realize that it would be precisely that — the last time like the one we had just shared, that I would have with my mother. December roses were gathered that day!

Joy still managed that first week in December to purchase my yearly Christmas tree ornament. She had begun several years ago to give me the ugliest ornament she could find for our tree! We laughed each year as she unveiled her "special" ornament for the year. I couldn't imagine anything uglier than the ones she had given me before: a very ugly Santa, a skinny cat (I'm not an animal lover, especially cats), and a silly alligator, to name a few. But this year took the cake — the largest plastic silver bell that she could find! I mean, this bell is hideous! It is about six inches in circumference and about eight inches in height — way too big to even be able to hide on the tree. Of course the boys thought it was great! I tried to put it behind the tree but each time the boys came in, they found it and placed it right out in front, much to Joy's delight! There would be a Christmas, and very soon, that I would lovingly look at each of those ornaments and have a wonderful memory, painful as it would be!

Carolyn and Mark had been going to Florida for the past two Christmases to be with their youngest daughter, Traci, and her husband Scott. This year was to be no exception. It made me feel a little sad not to have them here for Christmas, but I realized that was selfish. She needed to gather roses for her Decembers too!

I wanted my Christmas to stay the same as always but I knew it couldn't be that way forever. I was just sad to see what I was used to, slipping away. I missed our baby boys who would wake up very early Christmas morning and slip into bed together and giggle as Andrew read a Christmas story to Adam while waiting for the magical hour of 7:00 to wake us up so we could go downstairs to see what Santa had brought! They would run into our room and announce the time, "It's 7:00 o'clock." And then they would go into Nina's room to wake her up. Sitting at the top of the stairs, they would wait for Daddy to turn on the Christmas tree lights and have the camera ready. He would most always say, "Doesn't look like he's been here yet." They would nervously laugh and tell him they knew he was just kidding! Wasn't he?

If I close my eyes tightly, I can almost see their excited faces and candy apple cheeks as they entered the room and saw the gifts. They were always appreciative of each and every thing Santa had brought. If they were disappointed, they never showed it. What fun we had on those precious Christmas mornings! The lights, the candles, the smells in the kitchen and the love around that tree were memories that I will cherish forever. I had dozens and dozens of roses!

We would celebrate Christmas early with Carolyn and Mark and I would be happy that they were spending Christmas with their family, too. After all, Christmas isn't one day, is it? No! It can't be just one day, or I've lost the meaning again.

By now I know you clearly realize that I really don't like change at all — any type of change. But if one doesn't change, one doesn't grow. I had to face the realization that our children may want to start their own traditions some day (eek!) and that would be good. Really, it would! You see, Jim and I had done that and it was good — very good.

Many nights during the last few months of my mother's life, as she painfully struggled because of arthritis in her knees, to go upstairs each night for bed, I would walk behind her to keep her from falling. It usually was quite a long process. Instead of being frustrated at something she could not help, I began to spend that time looking at the boys pictures which adorned the stairwell and I would pray for them and their families. All their baby pictures and pictures of our family smiled back at me. Each picture reminded me of different phases of their boyhood days and how proud we are of the way they have grown, married wonderful Christian girls, and were beginning their own families.

No! Things will never be the same, but if we are blessed with grandchildren to hold and to love, there would be other memories to be made. I realize that I must let go of the past in order to embrace the future. Our family is blessed to have a past that is worth holding onto. For some people the past is very painful and not worth repeating. But for me, I would do it all over again and that is a very comforting thing to contemplate! I would have bouquets and bouquets of roses for many Decembers to come, as the Lord allowed!

I love Christmas! I wish I could go shopping with Sandy the way we have done so many years before. I feel so dependent. Why is that so hard for me to accept? A wheelchair! I never wanted to have a wheelchair. I know now why Nina gets frustrated sometimes when Sandy takes her shopping. People don't realize that when they want to stop and look at something, they can just do it. We have to yell at the person who's pushing us to stop so we can see! I never realized how difficult that could be until I found myself in the situation. But I won't complain too long. "Thank you, Lord, for giving me yet another Christmas. I love it so much!

Thank you, Lord, for loving me and for all of your blessings. Give me strength, Lord. I am weak when I am alone. Help me through what lies ahead for me. I cannot climb this mountain alone. Won't you heal me, Lord, please? I really want to be healed ... but if not, let me praise you through my cancer."

Chapter 26

Christmas Treasures

Sherry, our marketing coordinator from the publishing company, had become so dear to Joy and to me. She called me one day before Christmas and said that she wanted to visit us. We were so excited. She would be coming in February. It was something for Joy to look forward to. It would be a belated Christmas present for us. I thanked God for Sherry every day. She was so convinced that *To Run The Race With Joy* had the power to change lives with the message. She worked very hard to see that it was promoted even though she had many other authors to work with also. We could hardly wait to finally see her face to face. She had become like a sister to us.

On December 10, Joy took the chemotherapy Novatrone, her second treatment. Still she had no significant hair loss. She was so pleased! Debby and I had our coonskin caps ready and waiting just in case the hair got thin!

My plan was to bake cookies all day December 13, just like old times. Mother and Joy sat in the family room as I rattled around in the kitchen baking while our Christmas music played on the stereo. As I completed the first batch and was ready to place them into the oven, I turned around and both of them were sound asleep. Well, it wasn't what I had planned but I hummed the carols as I continued my baking, and praised God that at least they were with me and their sleep looked and sounded sweet.

The next day we were to sing in our Christmas cantata at church. Joy and I had been practicing with the choir for weeks. I was amazed that she could still sing with her weakened lungs! She loved the choir. I fought tears as I helped her struggle to the front of the church and assemble with the rest of the choir members. She sang her heart out beside me that Sunday morning. I looked out and saw my mother and remembered the many Christmases before when she had also sung beside me in the choir with her lovely alto voice lifted to the heavens. We always said that with the Christmas cantata, Christmas began. It was such a vivid reminder of the truth of the season. Never was it so real as this Christmas — never! My attitude had indeed changed and my heart was full of peace and the good tidings of great joy!

I truly felt that this would be Joy's last Christmas here on earth with us because she seemed so weak. We spent Christmas Eve (Jim, Mother, Joy and I) at Teri and Kevin's home. This was the first Christmas Eve that both of our boys were spending away from home — Julie and Andrew were at Julie's parents' home, and Adam and Rita were to be with Rita's parents. I was happy for Teri's invitation because the evening would have been a little lonely. I had told Teri to take lots of pictures this year because I really didn't think Joy could possibly hang on much longer. I could look at her and literally see her life slipping away. She could barely walk and she seemed to be getting tired of the fight — tired of pushing against a fortress that would not move. Her body was too broken to be mended except for a miracle that we all still prayed for. Her life had already been a miracle so we could truly ask for no more. I believed God's work in her was almost to an end, almost completed. I weep bitter tears as I write this because it will be painful to say goodbye. Why does it have to be so very painful?

With tears, Teri agreed to try to make this Christmastime special and take lots and lots of pictures. And that we did! It was a very wonderful time for us all. My mother enjoyed being in the company of Kevin's sweet mother and they had a great time together. Joy seemed so happy even with the noise that comes to a house at Christmas where a very rambunctious five-year-old and his very active little dog live! We left their home Christmas Eve knowing that Joy would bask in the light of the family time she had shared with all of them during this most special night of the year, for the entire Christmas season. Teri would tell me later that it was the best Christmas ever!

We drove home that evening and the four of us, alone for the first time without at least one of the boys, spent some quiet time together before saying goodnight. It was different without the kids but Jim and I had offered to one of God's children a special Christmas and that would give us many memories, many roses!

As we prepared for bed and I kissed Jim, Mom and Joy goodnight, I was reminded that the Father knew all about my melancholy feelings. He is acquainted with heartache. I could not be sad. I must rejoice! And as I snuggled into my pillow with Jim's arms safely around me, I was rejoicing.

I love that beautiful carol, "Come Thou Long Expected Jesus, born to set Thy people free." Why did He do that? He didn't have to. He didn't have to die. What love! We are His people. He was born to set us free. And some day we will be free — free from sorrow, pain, suffering, death and dying, and — separation. But I must live, if God chooses and if He hasn't finished His work in me. We must all endure until He has completed us. We must lose self-will and desire God's will. And this is the most difficult part, to delight in God's will. Psalm 40:8 says, *"I desire to do your will, O my God; your law is within my heart."*

He wants us to delight in His will. Joy once said that she believed we must love the cross that we take up daily. It is a hard thing to do when that cross is so painful. Only Christ can help us to love it! And I am convinced that when we learn to love the cross He asks us to bear, then we are truly happy!

God knew this was to be our last Christmas with my mother. How I wish I would have known when I went into her room that Christmas Eve to kiss her goodnight — how I wish I would have known. But God was even then preparing me to bear that cross when the time came. Although it would prove to be the most painful experience of my life, He would not leave me to face it alone! I'm still struggling with that cross to this day. The pain is still deep, still so very deep. I have a long way to go, but I'm so glad that my Lord goes with me.

Chapter 27

A Downward Spiral

With Christmas over, we wondered what the next year, 1998, would bring. How much more time did Joy have? Sometimes I just wish God would reveal things like that and then when I really think about it, I realize that He surely does know best; our Father knows best! The comfort is that He won't give us more than we can handle. He has promised us that. If we knew everything, where would the trust be?

An MRI was scheduled for Joy on January 27. Teri was scheduled to take her. It turned out to be a very, very long MRI. Both Teri and Joy were exhausted when it was finally over. We had no idea what the results would bring. We were scheduled to meet with the doctor to discuss the results on February 4.

Jim, Teri and I went with Joy to talk to Doctor Beveridge. I just knew by the way he entered the room that things were not good. However, I was completely shocked to hear him tell us that Joy had developed brain cancer and that there were six lesions that showed up on her brain! It was all we could do not to look at one another, for I just knew that as soon as Teri's eyes met mine, we would not be able to contain our tears.

Joy was to begin a new treatment immediately. Dr. Beveridge talked to us about the side effects and the possibility of perhaps having to place a plate into her brain in order to vehicle the chemotherapy. I was in so much shock that I really don't even remember much about that visit except for hearing those five words: **Joy, you have brain cancer!** Over and over again I heard those same words, brain cancer ... brain cancer. Through it all, even the prospect of brain surgery, Joy seemed undaunted.

129

Teri and I cried together once we were alone. The tears were free-flowing and bitter. "She's all the extended family I have," Teri cried, as we held onto each other. "I don't think I can live without her." I comforted her as best I could with my own heart breaking.

With the spirit that belongs only to Joy, she insisted that we go to choir practice that evening after supper. We sat next to each other as usual, but hard as I tried, I just couldn't seem to sing with very much gusto. "Just stop it!" she whispered in my ear. "Cheer up. You just have to. It will be all right. We can't let all these people down because we have to live what we believe." She made a funny face at me as she made a silly remark about something we had been talking about on the way to practice, and I was soon actually giggling when I should have been singing.

When practice was over and it was time for prayer requests, Joy told the choir about the brain cancer. A silence fell over the choir like nothing I've ever "heard" — a deadly silence. No one knew what to say. I don't know how I did it but I stood up and said, "Oh, don't worry at all about this latest diagnosis. Her brain is so very, very small that it doesn't mean anything. The cancer will be completely zapped in one radiation treatment."

The spell was immediately broken and Joy laughed loudest of all. Once again, it was laughter that had made the difference. She winked at me and held onto my hand as the choir prayed for her. There were some tears as we left that evening, but it was settled. God was already providing to us the strength we needed for this latest devastating development.

My devotion for that evening, February 4, asked us to look back at all our past experiences and think about how the Lord had led, and how to think upon the Lord's sufficiency. It was a perfect reminder of the Lord's faithfulness to us. *"For I am convinced that neither death nor life, neither angels nor demons, neither the present nor the future, nor anything else in all creation, will be able to separate us from the love of God that is in Christ Jesus our Lord"* (Romans 8:38, 39). We had to hold on to that wonderful promise, and we would.

I'm okay! I told Sandy and Teri that I am okay. I have brain cancer! I know I don't have much longer. I do all my best crying in the bathtub. Tonight was no exception. "I know, Lord, that you walk in my footsteps and you can't get much closer than that. But I don't want to lose my mind. I want to keep my dignity, Lord. Please! I don't want to be a burden on anyone."

When trials come, the question is not what happens to us; but what happens in us, not what kind of trials come to us, but our attitude towards them. That is what will count for eternity.

"We will soon have to tell the kids about the diagnosis and what it means. Lord, help them to accept your will — help me to accept it, Lord. You know that I long to be healed, but only if it is your will. I love you, Lord!"

Chapter 28

A Promised Gift From God

We were completely preoccupied with Joy's devastating report from the doctor. And then on February 5, I received word from my family in West Virginia that one of my mother's sisters, Mildred, had died. It was sudden and something that we did not expect. She was very close to my mother and therefore Mother took the news very hard. We made plans to go to West Virginia immediately.

My sister and I had spent summers as children with Mother's family in West Virginia. Her sisters were more like "mothers" to Carolyn and me. Each one (she had five in all) had her own special place in our hearts. I wept for the loss of that part of my childhood but I knew that Aunt Mimmie was with Jesus.

Mother decided to stay for an extra week after the funeral to be with her sister, Grayce, who had lived with Aunt Mimmie. I knew they would have a lot of crying to do together and a lot of healing to get through. It proved to be the best decision we could have made for both of them. They shared their last week on this earth together, just the two of them, although at the time, we didn't know it.

Once back in Virginia, cancer became the hot topic once again. Joy had her first radiation treatment on February 9. We told the kids at dinner that evening about her brain cancer. They became very quiet. But, because of the way Joy reacted to everything, she soon had them laughing through their tears. We vowed to pray harder than ever before.

Sherry's plans to visit were coming together — something to look forward to. We made plans to take her to lunch and for a little sightseeing trip even though we knew Joy would have to use the wheelchair. Joy knew that was a given.

Then a few days later, from out of the blue, Julie and Andrew announced to us that we were to become grandparents!! I can't even tell you the indescribable joy that filled my heart. Joy and I cried and screeched and carried on. Joy knew in her heart, she would tell me later, that she would never live to see the baby grow up, but all she asked was that God allow her to see the baby and love him for a little while. I also prayed that prayer over and over again.

God's timing is so incredibly perfect, He was already preparing that child to help heal our hearts that were to be broken much sooner than we could have imagined, much sooner!

Great grandmother Nina was delighted to hear the news as was Aunt Grayce. It would give them something else to focus on. Andrew had called them in West Virginia and he could tell that it was just the medicine they needed. The promise of new life — how could that not help but cheer a saddened heart!

With Joy finally realizing that she had to make plans to go on disability from work, and her acceptance of the wheelchair (well, almost an acceptance), and with her radiation underway, we looked forward to Sherry's visit and of course to the arrival in October of our baby.

Are you sure that some of you didn't hear very loud proclamations in your part of the country from here in Virginia on that February evening in 1998, announcing, *"I'm Going To Be A Grandma. I'm Going To Be A Grandma!!"* A prouder grandma there couldn't be! "Oh, Lord Jesus. You are so very faithful." How I needed this news just now, and just how much I would cherish it in the days to follow, I was yet to find out.

When I keep my mind on my circumstances, I begin to belly-ache and God doesn't like us to bellyache. I also begin to ask, "Why?" when I should be saying, "Why not me?"

His word says, "In everything give thanks," not just in the good things but in everything! "Lord, keep my mind off my circumstances, and keep it on Christ. Lord, let me live to see Andrew and Julie's baby. Let me love him, if only for a little while."

Chapter 29

Our Sherry

Mom came home from West Virginia, Sherry arrived, and life continued. Sherry looked wonderful and it was as though we had known her forever. She was surprised at Joy's failing appearance but still amazed at her spirit. Mom, though still grieving, was glad to be home again.

We spent the time with Sherry going out to lunch, sightseeing and dinner at Debby and Scott's home. We also celebrated my mother's 92nd birthday, and did a speaking engagement at our favorite church (other than our own, of course), Rose Hill Baptist. One of our favorite friends from Faith, Zelda Artz, came to Rose Hill with us. I also invited Mother for she had never heard me speak. We had a great evening with those wonderful ladies from Rose Hill. Sherry spoke, as did Joy and I, and we had a book-signing. It was nice for Sherry to see firsthand the results of some of the things that she had set up for us.

We also took Sherry to WAVA radio station in Rosslyn, Virginia, to meet Janet Parshall and to NBC to meet Willard Scott. She had her picture taken with them and was thrilled. She instantly knew why we loved Janet, and of course Willard was his lovable self, a big teddy bear!

Janet had Joy and me on her radio program *Janet Parshall's America*, in May of 1997 to discuss *To Run The Race With Joy*. We were on the air with her for an entire hour. She was very moved with Joy's testimony and our ministry. Willard had written comments that appear on the front cover of that book.

Sherry and I went with Joy for another brain scan. We stood beside Joy and watched as they laid her on the metal table and prepared her for the scan. We laughed with her as we took pictures. Once she was inside the machine, we had to leave. We could see her through a window just outside of the room. I noticed a microphone nearby and I asked the nurse if we could talk to Joy over the microphone. "Not just yet," she said, "but when the scan is over, I'll turn it on and you can talk to her."

Sherry looked at me with that "What do you have on your mind now?" look and I motioned for her to come close to the microphone with me. As Joy was coming out from the machine the nurse told me I could start speaking when she flipped the button. When she was completely out, I said, "Look, Sherry, her brain is really very, very small. See it?"

Joy raised up and looked very puzzled for a split second before she realized what we had done. We all cracked up! She didn't think we could even see her let alone talk to her. No one had ever talked to her before over the microphone! The technicians were in stitches. "Only you would think of that, Sandy," Joy retorted. "Very funny."

We laughed a lot during those days with Sherry. We would see her again, the two of us, but under different circumstances — very different circumstances!

I love Sherry. God sent her to us, of that I am sure. She is a special person and like a sister. I only wish I had more time on this earth with her.

She wrote a beautiful poem for me. I cried when I read it. It has touched my heart in a way she will never know:

A Testimony For All Time

As we walk down life's pathway, not knowing where it
*   will lead,*
Trusting in God, to meet all our needs,
How often we forget that He knows best,
When storm clouds gather and we are put to the test.
But, when I see your faith so strong and true,
It's plain to see God's love and strength in you.
Although there may come a tear to your eye,
You look to God for your strength and never ask why.
You never seem to complain,
As you trust in God to heal your pain.
You have given us a glimpse of God's grace;
We see His peace as we look upon your face.
Some things in life we will never understand;
But God is in control and for each life there is a plan.
You may think your life is too short to do God's will,
And His plan you will not fulfill.
I would like to assure you that you have not failed,
For you have run your race well.
We see Christ in you and in your life his mercy shines,
And your story of faith will be a testimony for all time.

Sherry Neuenschwander, 1998

Chapter 30

How Much More, Lord?

It was at the end of February that Joy became convinced that she could not continue to go to work any longer. The trip to Washington was too far and she could not drive it! Also, her decreasing stamina prevented her from doing much of anything beyond just getting there. NBC sent tapes home to her and set her up with an office so she could continue to work at her leisure, but from home. It worked pretty well for a little while but that, too, became almost an impossibility as her strength continued to dwindle. It certainly was good for her morale not to have to just abruptly quit work altogether and for that I praised God!

We spent the month of March doing some book-signings, chemotherapy, radiation and trips (as many as we could fit in) to Bethany Beach. We were scheduled to go to New York to speak at a women's retreat at the Goodwill Evangelical Presbyterian Church the end of the month. We were very excited. We had met some of those wonderful women when we conducted our Presbytery retreat the previous year and we were anxious to renew acquaintances with them once again.

We had arranged to speak at Cornerstone Chapel in Leesburg, Virginia, on the night of March 12. Teri and Debby went with us and we had a great time except for the fact that Teri's car broke down. God certainly provided though. A most generous woman, I believe her name was Ann, willingly offered to drive us all the way home. Now, from our home in Alexandria, that would be about an hour each way. We praised God for her and for His provision. She will never know how much that personally meant to me. I didn't realize just how much until I arrived home.

I was met at the door by my longtime dear friend, Barbara Jesser, who had come from Charlottesville, Virginia with her husband, Bill, to spend the weekend with us. My mother, she told me, had been taken to the hospital with what appeared to be a stroke. Jim was there with her. Debby took me over the hospital right away and for the next several hours, Mother's condition seemed to be very serious. We feared the worst.

She was admitted to the hospital and was put into the intensive care unit. However, Mom improved dramatically over the next few days and was released from the hospital just five days later. With my sister's help in staying with her, Joy, Jim and I went to New York as we had planned. Mom looked very well and her speech and coordination were almost back to normal the day we left. I praised God. I just never expected her to be anything else except "normal." This was just a little setback. After all, she was my mother and I would have her for at least a few more years, if not forever!!

We had a marvelous time in New York. I was especially glad to have Jim along. While Joy and I conducted the retreat, Jim and the pastor, Stuart Pohlman, hung around together all weekend. On Sunday morning, Joy and I as well as Jim were asked to address the congregation. It was such a blessed weekend. The spirit of God truly was present.

It was there that we met Dr. Louise Nielsen, who has been such a blessing to me personally. She became like my sister that weekend. It was only the grace of God that brought her to that retreat and her experience there changed her life forever. I hope I have adequately expressed my gratitude to her in the opening pages of this book for all the support and encouragement she has been to me with Joy and in the publication of this book.

Our return to Virginia found my mother even more improved and things were quite back to "normal." She seemed much like her old self again. I was encouraged. Joy was tired from our trip but she also seemed to be doing well.

Then one evening shortly after we came back from New York, Joy had an accident in her car. We had been telling her for weeks that she had to stop driving but she wouldn't listen to us. She had her foot on the accelerator thinking it was the brake (because of the fact she had very little feeling in her right foot and leg) and she went backwards all the way down our street. Thankfully, she didn't get hurt nor did she hurt anyone else. She did damage to our neighbor's mailbox as well as a parked car, but that was the extent of it. Shortly afterwards, she willingly gave up driving. It was the hardest thing she had to do. It broke my heart to think of her having to sell her little yellow bumblebee, but she knew it was just a matter of time before that would happen. For now, she just looked at it when we picked her up or took her home and she started it up every few days. The time would come to sell but not just yet! More and more she had to rely on others. It was apparent to everyone that it was killing her!

"Oh, Lord," I prayed, "give her understanding and give her the ability to relinquish yet more of her independence. May we have the wisdom to help her, while allowing her to keep her dignity and her spirit. There is a fine line, Lord. Help us to listen to you as you lead."

I am confident He will not give us more than we can bear for He has promised. I look back at the trials we have been through and the wonderful way He has delivered us and I know He is faithful. I draw upon those past answers to prayer now, and when I put everything into perspective, I ask Him to forgive me for asking, "How much more?" He is indeed my Shepherd and I am His sheep. I must rest in that.

"So many things to ask you for, Lord! Nina's stroke was not expected at all. Sometimes we ask, 'Why?' Lord, and I know we should not do that. Sandy doesn't need anything else on her plate now, Jesus. I thank you for loving me when I am not lovable at all and when I question you. I ask that you heal Nina, Lord. Let her know your peace and quiet Sandy's spirit.

I have to stop working now and it was a hard decision to come to. I can't drive over to Washington every day. I get there and I'm so tired I can't get anything done once I'm there. Some days I don't even feel like going to work at all! Thank you, Lord, that Mr. Russert has okayed having an office set up for me at home. I know they are doing this for me, but I promise I'll work whenever I'm able. How did it come to this? So many changes and so fast.

I had an accident in my car tonight, Lord! It was so scary and I know I am going to have to give up driving but I honestly don't feel like that was my fault. I thought my foot was on the brake and it was on the gas!! Stupid! Anyone could have done that! Yet, I know Sandy and Teri will tell Dr. Beveridge and he will tell me to stop driving. They just don't realize what that will do to me. You know Lord, and so I'll just have to turn it over to you. So many trials — I'm so tired — can't even drag myself to bed some nights. I still cry in the bathtub but you know that. Tell my mom that I love and miss her! And be with Teri and Sandy and thank you that they are with me."

Chapter 31

Darkness Is Closing In

Easter, 1998, and we were spending it at the beach. Andrew and Julie were at Julie's parents for Easter dinner and we had Adam and Rita, Mother and Joy with us. We had never celebrated Easter there before, but my spring break usually falls the week before Easter so we took advantage of the time and decided to stay over for the Easter weekend. Mother had spent a few days with Carolyn and her family and they brought her to the beach on the Wednesday before Easter.

We had a good time that week, and Mom as well as Joy seemed to be doing well. One night we took everyone out to dinner at a nice restaurant overlooking the bay and my mother was thrilled. She kept telling me how nice the place was. We all had seafood, which we love, and Mom and I shared a large order of one of our favorite foods, hushpuppies! It was a memorable time.

Mom took us all for ice cream one night and she got her favorite, a strawberry sundae. She loved to treat everyone from time to time, and it made her feel good to do so. Her income was small and fixed but it was important for her to be able to do something like that once in a while. We laughed at the large ice cream sundae that Adam ordered and ate. Mom seemed very happy. Joy said she felt sick and opted not to go out with us that evening so she had stayed at home. I loved Joy but sometimes I had to admit it was nice for just "us" to go out. I hope that wasn't a selfish thought and God knows my heart, but sometimes I felt smothered by so much dependence and so much care-giving. Do any of you understand what I am saying? Does it make any sense at all? I wouldn't change my life but when you can't breathe, you can't live. Sometimes I just needed to be able to breathe. That night, I felt as though I could breathe for a while!!

We left on Easter Sunday afternoon to go back to Virginia. I sat in back with Mom and it's funny but I can't remember much about the trip except that I covered her hands as she slept, because the car seemed too cool and I was concerned that she might be cold. I fussed over her to get her comfortable as I placed a pillow beneath her head.

Once home, we unpacked the car and after I had put everything away, I got a glass of iced tea and Joy and I went out front to sit on the porch. Mother was in her chair talking to my sister on the phone. All of a sudden I heard a crash and my mother called out my sister's name. I ran into the house to find my mother on the floor. She had attempted to walk without her walker or her cane, from her chair into the kitchen while carrying things in both hands. She seemed disoriented but she knew everyone and she knew where she was. I was so aggravated at her for walking without her cane that I'm afraid I was less than sweet at first. I had told her **over** and **over** and **over** and **over** again not to walk without the walker or cane but she was stubborn and convinced at times that she did not need either. This was one of those times.

I got her into a chair and called her doctor. He suggested that unless she couldn't walk and since the pain was focused in the area of her tailbone, that we just use Tylenol and observe her for a while. The emergency room of the hospital was full and overflowing and he didn't want her to have to wait the long hours that he knew it would take until she could be seen. I was to call his office on Monday morning. Joy looked tired and I knew she needed to get home, so after getting Mother upstairs and into bed, I helped Joy to the car, and Jim drove her home.

Mom slept fairly well Sunday night and as I had previously arranged for a full time companion to be with her Monday, I went to work. I checked on her throughout the day and even though she was very sore from the fall, she seemed okay. When I got home in the afternoon, she was sleeping. She ate dinner in her room because I knew for a few days the steps would be a problem. I sat with her as she ate her dinner and we talked. With her current state of depression I had to assure her over and over that it would take more than a few days to get herself back to where she had been physically and she would be fine again. I truly believed that, even though her usual response to most things was negative. I didn't realize that in the next few hours everything would change in my family forever — everything!

I should have known something was wrong when she called me in the middle of the night and she seemed disoriented. That wasn't really too unusual because sometimes she was that way, but as I helped her to the bathroom she seemed to be much weaker in her knees and I had trouble getting her on the toilet seat. Jim came and helped me and we got her back into bed. I gave her two Tylenol tablets and tried to get her as comfortable as I could. I kissed her goodnight and told her I loved her as I usually did every night.

It had been a very stressful ordeal, more so than usual. As I fell back into bed I just closed my eyes and said, "Lord, I can't do this anymore." Why did I pray that prayer? I've asked myself a hundred times over. It seemed that with Joy's worsening condition and then this additional problem with Mom, that I, once again, felt that I couldn't breathe. But I didn't want an answer in the way it came. I didn't want it at all.

I slept an extra hour the next morning because of the stress I had encountered during the night. I just couldn't get up when the alarm went off at 6:20. Every bone in my body ached and I felt my heart palpitations stronger than ever.

When I went into Mom's room to get her up and ready for the day, I found her in a very confused and dazed condition and lying in a pool of green liquid. She reached up with a fearful look in her eyes and touched my face but no words would come.

My whole world stopped! In that instant when her eyes met mine, my world stopped. That look told me she knew she would never come back to our home again! With a cold fear gripping my heart, I called the rescue squad. As I heard the sirens in the background the darkness began to envelop me and again, I found it hard to breathe. I heard myself praying for the strength that I knew was only a whisper away!

147

We had a good time Easter at the beach. I'm just the happiest when I am there. "Thank you, Lord, for dying for me and for loving me in spite of my attitude which is sometimes not the greatest and in spite of my continual sinful nature!"

Sandy called me this morning and told me that Nina had another stroke and is in the hospital. "Oh, Lord, she sounded so scared — I know how she feels. Losing a mom is just the hardest thing to do. I want to be with her, Lord, but I am so weak and so tired. Help me to be able to be there for her as she was for me when my own mother was in the hospital for so long before you took her.

The boys will be so devastated, Lord. They love their Nina so much. Be with them, Lord, and comfort Nina at this time and give her peace that you are with her. Lord, you hold our lives in your hands. You have all the answers and in your own time you will reveal them to us. Help us to wait upon you."

Chapter 32

Hearts Begin To Break

I had never ridden in an ambulance before. The siren sounds so much louder when you are the one racing for help. People wouldn't move over so the ambulance could pass. "Why won't they move?" I frantically cried to the driver.

"We face this all the time," he replied. "I just don't understand it myself. But don't worry we are making good time."

I decided then and there that I would move to the right immediately the next time I was driving and heard a siren. Never again would I be impatient because I had to stop for a rescue vehicle. Your whole perspective changes when it becomes personal.

I prayed the whole way to the hospital for the Lord to spare Mother until I could calm her down, quiet her fears and tell her I loved her. I just couldn't bear the thought that I might have to remember the last time I saw her face as I had seen it just a few minutes before.

Once at the hospital, I knew Jim was only minutes away and that he had called Carolyn. The minutes seemed like hours as I waited alone in that waiting room. I couldn't find out any information, and the longer I sat there, the more frantic I became. Just like so many times before, I couldn't breathe. I felt my very breath going from my body.

Jim and Carolyn arrived, as did Mark. I was no longer alone. I thanked God for my family. Carolyn and I were allowed to see Mom but she looked terrible and very frightened. We hoped she understood us as we tried to comfort and soothe her. She tried to communicate with us but could not. I left the room for just a few minutes to give Jim and Mark an update and to tell them she was going to have a CAT scan performed. I had no sooner delivered the information when a nurse hurriedly came to get me. Mom had suffered a seizure. Carolyn was almost hysterical. I thought it was the end as they ushered us just outside her room so they could work on her. We held each other and prayed.

Mother calmed down after being given medication. The scan revealed a huge blood clot in the left side of her brain and numerous clots on the right side. It was a touch-and-go situation. They could really tell us nothing. Time! It would just take time. But they told us it didn't look good at all; the clot was just too large! A neurosurgeon would be called in and her primary care doctor was on her way.

The guilt I felt was overwhelming. If I'd only taken her to the emergency room on Sunday night, if I hadn't been so aggravated with her over not using her walker and cane, if I had been more observant when I had gotten up with her at 3:00 that morning. What if... what if! She had become very difficult the last few months. Her depression was killing all of us and I had been so frustrated and so stressed. Joy's condition was deteriorating, my temper had been short and I could fix nothing, nothing at all! And now this!! The darkness was almost unbearable and I could see no light now, none at all.

My heart raced and my body felt numb as we waited for them to move Mother to the intensive care unit of the hospital. I called Andrew, Adam and Joy, and Carolyn called her daughters, Kim and Traci. I really didn't think she would live through the day.

For the next 48 hours Mom hovered between life and death. We spent almost every waking hour with her. It was heart-wrenching to hear our boys whisper to her of their love as their tears fell upon her soft porcelain face. They loved her so. She had lived with us almost their whole lives and she was as much a part of them as we were.

After discussion with the neurosurgeon, we decided not to have her go through brain surgery to remove the clot. It was very, very dangerous surgery and given her age, she would likely not make it off the operating table. We also opted, through many tears, to have her listed once again as a "No Code." It was undoubtedly the best decision under the circumstances, but very difficult to make!

Mom was admitted to the hospital on Tuesday, April 14, and up until Thursday, April 16, she wakened only minutes at a time and not very often. We talked to her constantly when we were with her, which was almost every minute of the day, and told her we loved her. Her heart beat was strong and I felt for a while that she may yet make another remarkable recovery. I prayed for that. They even moved her out of the intensive care unit. Surely this was a good sign.

Joy was undergoing her chemo and various tests while trying to support me as best she could. I knew I had to devote all my time to my mother and she wanted me to do that, but all the same I felt torn. "Lord, I'm only one person. Please give me wisdom." Joy felt that I was spending too much time at the hospital and I know she was thinking of me, but I was angry because a part of me felt that even in the face of death, Joy was still just a little jealous of the time I spent with my mother. Oh, understand, my mother was also a little jealous of the time I spent with Joy. I had felt like a rubber band much of the time over the years. No matter how much I tried to talk to each of them about the struggles of the other one, and given the fact that I knew they loved each other and the Lord, I always felt as though I couldn't bridge the gap that seemed to grow larger between them with each passing day. I was in the middle and no matter which way I turned, to one of them, I had turned the wrong way. Now, I felt as though I had devoted too much time to Joy and not enough time to my mother, for here she was dying and Joy was very much alive, albeit, very sick!

This was my mother! It had been easier in a way to deal with Joy's cancer because it was physical. Mom's depression was emotional and very hard to deal with. I hadn't tried hard enough and now I would not have another chance to try! My heart was breaking! It was the worse pain I have ever felt in my whole life! I hoped my friends were praying for me because I could not pray for myself. I didn't feel worthy to pray. I had let my mother and the Lord down. For the first time in my life, I felt lost and darkness threatened to consume me.

Nina is no better. Sandy looks very tired and I told her she is spending too much time at the hospital, but I know how she feels because I did that when my own mother was in for so long a time. I guess I never did spend as much time as Sandy and Carolyn do with Nina, but people are different. I was so sick when my mother was in the hospital. I couldn't be there because of all the treatments and the appointments I had to go to. It's always been difficult for me to spend a lot of time in the hospital but I want to support Sandy.

"Help me, Lord, and give me strength to help Sandy and her family. I feel lonely when I can't be with them. I feel like I'm not normal. I think it is the separation that is the most painful. Thank you for Chip and for Teri and her family. I know you have placed so many people in my life and I love you so much for that."

Chapter 33

Our God Reigns

I slept very little during those first four days. My heart seemed to be in constant prayer and yet I didn't feel as if I could pray at all. I felt so unworthy! I went through the motions of life as I struggled in my spirit. I spent every minute at my mother's bedside, singing to her and holding her hand. Carolyn and I bathed her, changed her, washed her hair, and tried to keep her as we knew she would have wanted had she known anything at all.

I called our brothers. David made arrangements to come to Virginia. I could not reach Bill, who lives in California. I prayed she would awaken long enough to recognize Dave, for I knew it would mean so much to him. I prayed she would awaken to recognize me just once more. I begged God for that when I could pray and make any sense at all.

Pastor Neil, who visited often, told me to tell her that I loved her as often as I could and to pray to the Lord that He would allow her to hear me. That helped, and I did just that all the time!

I felt overcome with grief and I cried until I felt I could cry no more. My heart literally hurt with the deepest agony I had ever felt. Jim would hold me at night as I lay sobbing. He didn't even need to talk to me, it was just a comfort to have him hold me. His mother had gone to be with the Lord in 1974 so he could empathize with me. I knew he was praying for me.

On Thursday morning, the fourth day, as I was getting ready to go to the hospital, Jim's long-time secretary, Patty Upshaw, whom I have loved like a sister, came and ministered to me. She had been so sweet to my mother for many years, and knew our family well. Her husband is pastor of the Rose Hill Baptist Church and we consider

153

them dear friends. She prayed with me and asked me to recount the many wonderful memories my mother had shared with me, with our boys and our family. She was very aware of the recent difficult times but she reminded me that it was Satan, the father of lies, who was trying to erase a multitude of precious memories by replacing those memories with a few isolated incidents of misunderstanding, so small when compared to a lifetime. She sweetly reminded me that Satan wanted to rob me of those blessings and I just couldn't let him do that.

We cried together and for the first time since my mother had been hospitalized, I could see a ray of light in my darkened world. I will cherish her ministry to me forever. I spent the day at the hospital singing to Mom as usual, but I kept remembering all the wonderful times we had spent together — the birthdays, anniversaries, vacations, weddings, holidays, the boys' recitals, concerts, plays and ball games, meals we had prepared and eaten together, picnics, laughter and tears we had shared, things we had prayed together about, all the things that make up a loving and godly family. They were enough to keep me praising God the whole time I was with her. I even wrote them down as they were brought to my remembrance. I couldn't recount all of them for they were too numerous. A lot of those wonderful memories included Joy, and I remembered their love for each other. I knew that when it was all said and done, they would remember that too!

Jim had to go out of town to court that day and was to be gone overnight. Joy spent the night with me and when she went upstairs to prepare for bed, I decided that I needed to have some very private and quiet time with the Lord. I wanted to make a confession to Him and I needed to be alone.

As I went to Him in real prayer for the first time in a good many days, the tears were free-flowing. I read my devotions and I was blessed beyond measure. It dealt with our soul's conflicts. We must wrestle with our sin and take it to God, confess it and accept His forgiveness and then let it go. But that must be done with God alone.

I confessed to Him and asked His forgiveness for all the things I had done and the sharp and sometimes unfeeling things I had said to my mother during the last few difficult months. Even though I had confessed those things to Him almost as soon as I had said them, I needed to do it again, once and for all. I then asked God to forgive my mother for unkind things that she had also done even though I knew that she had confessed those things to Him as I had. She often told me, usually when I went in each night to kiss her before she went to sleep, that she knew she had gotten short-tempered and she was sorry. We never went to bed angry at each other, and we told each other, "I love you," every night of our lives. It was as though we each found ourselves frustrated and not knowing what to do, and we were both searching for the same thing, wisdom and understanding of her depression.

And then I asked God that she remember only the love we shared, for it was far stronger and far greater than the depression. I wanted her to remember the bond we had together — I wanted to remember that also!

After I had confessed and poured out my heart to the Lord and I was completely exhausted, I asked the Lord for one more thing, that He allow her to open her eyes, recognize me and hear me tell her that I loved her, just one more time before He took her home! Nevertheless, I would accept His will for her life. I felt I had asked for the most impossible thing in the world but I boldly asked for it nevertheless. His word tells us in Psalm 37:4 that He will give us the desires of our heart and that is what I asked for. *"Delight yourself in the Lord and he will give you the desires of your heart."* As tears poured down my cheeks and onto the picture that I had been holding of Mom and me in happier days, I knew that whatever God chose to do concerning my request, I was at peace.

As I went upstairs, Joy and I prayed together, and I slept well for the first time in over four days.

The next morning as I arrived in Mom's room expecting to try once again, as I had every other morning, to awaken her, I was absolutely amazed to see that her eyes were wide open. I threw my things on the chair and rushed over to her and took her hands in mine. I said to her "Mom, do you know who I am?"

She very plainly said, "Of course. You are Sandy."

I could hardly contain myself as I hugged and kissed her and said to her, "That is right. Do you know I love you very much?"

She looked right into my eyes and said the words that I will remember as long as I live even though I had heard them many times before. "Yes. And I love you too!" Those words never sounded sweeter than they did then. She focused on my face for a few seconds, closed her eyes, yawned a very big yawn, immediately fell into a deep sleep and slept the rest of the day like she had never slept before!

God had given me the desire of my heart and more. I praised Him. God let the tears wash down my face unashamedly as the nurses came and went. I called Jim as soon as I knew he was back in town to tell him what had happened. I could hardly wait to tell everyone what God had done. My wonderful friend, Zelda, came into the room a short time later and rejoiced with me over God's marvelous love. She had been such a support to me. I counted on her and she never let me down. I knew she prayed for me when I could not pray for myself. I let my tears wash down her face and neck as she held me in her arms while she once again prayed for our Father's comfort.

I called Joy at her house and my sister who had to go to work that day, and let them know that Mom had opened her eyes for just a little bit and what had happened.

Carolyn usually relieved me in the evenings for a while on the days she could not be with me. She is a nurse and teaches in an LPN program. Unfortunately her year was closing and her students were preparing for final exams and graduation. I knew she was torn between her obligations to them and her desire to be with me, but there was really nothing she could do. Mom was holding her own and we saw to it that one of us was with her almost constantly. Many of our friends came to be with me during the day, and of course Jim, the boys and Julie and Rita were with me as much as they could be. I could always count on one of them or the pastor or dear Zelda, to come just when I needed someone the most. God seemed to work it out perfectly. Our family and the family of God are wonderful!

I kept Carolyn posted throughout the day. At the end of the school day, she would make the 30-45 minute trip to the hospital and be there until late at night. Alone with Mom in the evenings, I knew that she had her own private talks with God and her own tears of grief. I knew she talked to Mom just as I did during the day. It was a shared grief but grief that we each had to handle alone with God and with our mother.

I didn't realize it that day, but we would have to continue this for three very long weeks. God's grace and strength had just begun to work in our lives!

Jim had to go to Charlottesville and I spent the night with Sandy. We went out to a pizza place for dinner but I couldn't eat. I felt so nauseous. I hated to tell her but just after we ordered I knew I had to leave and go home. It is a terrible feeling. We took the pizza to go and it was all I could do to get to the car. I cried as I sat in the tub that night (my usual place to cry). I am so very weak and I feel so tired. "I want to be healed, Lord. I really want to be healed — but not my will."

Sandy came up to bed and I could tell that she had been crying also. We cried and prayed together — and we talked.

Tears do help. Especially when you are crying with a friend and you are praying with them, your hearts seem to be as one in the Lord. "Help me, Lord, to be a better prayer warrior for you."

Chapter 34

Where Do Broken Hearts Go?

There is a rock and roll song titled "Where Do Broken Hearts Go?" My heart was breaking a little more each day and the only place I knew to go, the only place where I could even hope to find comfort, was to my Savior. And to Him I went almost constantly. Without Him, I could not even imagine the despair I would feel nor the hopelessness. I drew upon His strength moment to moment.

Joy and I had been scheduled to conduct a women's retreat for a local Methodist church the first weekend in May. I had put off canceling it because I kept hoping Mother would improve but I was only kidding myself. I talked to Joy and made the phone call to the retreat coordinator, Judy Schulman, and let her know. She assured me that they would be able to find another speaker and she also assured me of their prayers. In the months to come she became a dear friend to me and to Joy as she helped transport Joy to and from her appointments, or came just to be her companion.

Each day in that hospital brought more and more pain. Mother developed pneumonia as her temperature soared, and the brain surgery that the neurosurgeon had thought might be possible when Mother's heart beat continued to strengthen, was cancelled. She had to endure feeding tubes and her hands were swollen beyond belief because of the IV's. We bathed her face and body in cold compresses, changed her diapers and turned her from side to side every hour to keep her as comfortable as we could. We were told to try to arrange a nursing home for her as soon as possible, for it appeared that she might linger on in this state for some time!

It had been my worst fear — a nursing home. How I had assured her so many times before that no matter how tough things got, I would never place her in a nursing home — never! And now here I was calling to arrange a conference with the administrator of a nearby nursing home. I could hardly get the words out when I made that phone call. But I realized that she needed far too extensive care for us to handle. Carolyn was almost hysterical when we discussed it. "I'm a nurse and I will not place her in one of those facilities! I will do it myself!"

Jim and I tried to make her see how impossible that would be for it already was taking the two of us plus round-the-clock nurses, to care for Mother. Physically, emotionally and financially we could not do that. She finally very reluctantly agreed and I made that phone call.

The day before our meeting at the nursing home, Mother took a turn for the worse. Her breathing became very labored, the pneumonia wasn't responding to medication and both of her lungs were affected. Her temperature continued to soar and she could not be moved, at least not in the near future. Part of me was relieved and part of me knew what that meant.

She had only awakened once or twice in the last week and only one time did I feel she knew us. She looked at Carolyn and me with a very curious look. "Do you know who we are?" I asked her. She blinked her eyes. "How many children do you have?" I continued.

"Four," she replied very clearly.

"Who am I?"

"My girl."

"Who am I?" Carolyn inquired.

"My girl," she stated.

"Who is David?" I then continued.

"Son-in-law."

Well, that was not exactly right but she knew he was in the family.

"Who is Bill?"

"Son-in-law!" she said in a faint voice. Then she closed her eyes once more and slept again like she was exhausted. That was the last time she spoke.

Of course, every time she even opened her eyes for just a few seconds, we told her we loved her, where she was and that we were

160

with her. One of us sang or talked to her most of the time we were with her. I didn't want her to be able to hear and only hear silence.

The boys would come and go and each time you could see the pain in their eyes and almost feel the heaviness of their breaking hearts. I thanked God that they, too, knew where broken hearts go. Julie and Rita came and went and their pain was also very obvious as they gently stroked Nina's cheek and helped us care for her.

We were now going into the second week. Mom was placed on morphine to keep her comfortable. She was just literally existing. I could tell even when her eyes were opened that she was not really alive. I just hoped that if she could at least hear me, she would hear words of love and comfort and songs of praise and peace. I ended each day with "Tis So Sweet To Trust In Jesus." I think I sang it as much for me as I did for her, it comforted me so. It was salve for my breaking heart!

Chapter 35

The Burden Grows Greater

Joy had received platelets on April 22 and things had not gone well at all. She broke out in a rash and she was very sick. I felt torn between wanting to be with her and needing to be with Mom. I called Rita and she offered to go and stay with Joy and take dinner to her. I was so grateful for Rita's willingness to do that. Joy simply had to eat. She weighed only 118 pounds. In 1991 when she was first diagnosed with cancer, she weighed 220. Her weight has gone down dramatically just in the last few weeks. She simply pushed the food around on her plate most of the time.

In times past, Joy and I would have spent these trying times together. When Jim was hospitalized several years ago, when my mother had her various surgeries throughout the years, when Adam was so sick in 1996, during Joy's mother's battle with cancer — all those times, we cried together, prayed together and supported one another, and now she was too sick to be with me in my darkest hour and I knew it was ripping her heart out!

I began to think that I might be losing both of them at the same time because Joy sounded so weak and so sick. I knew I couldn't entertain that thought for too long. God would have to take over for me because I felt my strength leave my body each night when I fell into bed; however, the next morning I found God had renewed me for yet another day. It could only have been strength from Him. I prayed for Him to keep Joy and be to her what I could not be for a while.

The very next day, through protests, Joy made her way to the hospital and struggled in obvious great pain to sit with me by Mom's bedside. She stayed holding Mother's hand for quite some time before Teri came to take her home. I noted tears in her eyes as she hugged me before she left. She felt she had let me down because she couldn't be with me all the time. She would never know how much her sacrifice had meant to me, for it took all the strength she could gather for her to make that trip.

That evening as I sat by Mom's bedside singing to her, my eyes were drawn to our hands. Mom's hand was covering my hand. My hand looked so very tiny under her hand, now so grossly enlarged from the fluids and the countless blood tests she had endured for the past two weeks. A casual observer might capture the picture through that small window as that of a mother comforting her child until he would draw back and see the whole picture and then realize that no! it was the mother, now a child, being comforted by a child, who had become the mother. And yet, I felt so strangely comforted by her hand covering mine.

As I sat there, my eyes still focused on our hands, childhood memories flooded my mind. I heard her voice and felt her soothing hands comforting me as she had so many times before when as a child I had hallucinated from having high fevers. I could almost hear her voice saying, "It's all right, honey. I'm here! You're only having a dream. I'll stay with you." I could almost feel her gentle and loving hands as she bathed my body, burning up with fever, with cool water. Many times she would stay by my bedside all night long until my fever broke.

Mother could only in recent years use the words, "I love you," freely. She had a difficult time putting her feelings into words. Yet I needed only to remember those special childhood times to know that she loved me. Her love had been very evident, just not spoken. I marveled at her ability to shower her grandchildren with lots of hugs and kisses and the affirmation, "I love you." Sometimes it made me jealous. But perhaps she had learned to do that from living in our loving home for so many years. Perhaps that was where she learned to demonstrate love because our home is full of love, hugs and kisses. "I love you" is said many times a day even though our boys are grown and have families of their own. What a marvelous tradition! Mom and I never failed to tell one another, "I love you," each and every night. We always ended every phone call with those words.

164

And so as I slipped my hand from beneath hers and prepared to leave for the evening, I seemed to feel renewed strength, perhaps from her love.

> *Tis so sweet to trust in Jesus,*
> *just to take Him at His word.*
> *Just to rest upon His promise,*
> *just to know thus saith the Lord.*
> *Jesus, Jesus how I trust Him,*
> *how I've proved him o'er and o'er.*
> *Jesus, Jesus, precious Jesus,*
> *Oh for grace to trust Him more.*

Louisa M.R. Stead

I went to the hospital today to sit with Nina. I held her hand and I remembered my own mother. I feel so sorry for Sandy.

Nina and I haven't always seen eye to eye. I've told Sandy that she knows how to pull her "chain" sometimes. And maybe I'm right but I probably shouldn't have said that. Sandy would get mad at me (of course she never stayed mad!) and she has told me that I haven't always been fair to her mother and maybe she is right. But I love Nina just the same. I told Sandy once that I loved Nina more than she realized but I don't know if she believed me or not. Nina is stubborn sometimes but then I *know* that I am. We both have had deep needs over the last few years and we certainly have not been ourselves, either one of us. God knows that. And we both depend too much on Sandy but then Nina is her mother and I know her first obligation is to her. Sandy told me that once, in love, and I accepted that and I knew it was right. But I thank God that she and Jim always take time for me, too. They include me in everything just like family and I know that at times it has been a difficult thing to do, but they have done it for me and with a lot of love.

"I thank you for Nina and for her love for you, Lord. Keep her free from fear of death. I feel afraid sometimes, too. Help us not to fear. Help me to be there for Sandy."

Chapter 36

He Giveth More Grace

My brother, David, arrived and I believe Mother may have recognized him, for her eyes opened briefly as he spoke with her. His heart was breaking too. He suffers from Parkinson's disease and panic attacks and I knew the trip in itself was difficult for him, let alone seeing our mother this way. As yet, we had not been able to contact my brother Bill, who lives in California. He was away on a trip and so we had to leave a message for him to call us as soon as he got home.

David stayed with us for several days. There was nothing he could do and Mother's condition remained the same. We both knew it would be only a little while until he would return. He kissed Mother goodbye with tears in his eyes, knowing he would not see her on this earth again. With a heavy heart, he flew back to Florida.

Carolyn's daughter, Kim, and her granddaughter, Amber, arrived from New Jersey and spent time with their grandmother caressing her tenderly and telling her of their love for her. Carolyn's younger daughter, Traci, who lives in Florida, had just spent several days with her grandmother the week before Easter and we advised her not to come home just yet because Nina really didn't recognize anyone now and she had spent really quality time with her when it had counted only a few weeks before. We kept her informed of Mother's condition on a daily basis.

By the beginning of the third week, April 27, the doctors were telling us that the time was very short and that we could have Hospice come in. It was the best decision we could have made. Carolyn and I met with the Hospice intake nurse on April 29 and arrangements were made to have Mother moved to a hospice room in the hospital.

We celebrated Andrew's birthday on April 28 but as hard as we tried, the celebration was difficult because Nina wasn't there. I bought a card for Andrew and signed Nina's name to it because if she had known I had not done that, she would have been very angry with me. I even included a small check in it as she would have done. Andrew had been very thankful that the Lord had not called his grandmother home on his birthday. He could not bear the thought that each year afterwards, he would have to remember that she had died on that day. A little thing maybe, but God had honored that simple prayer from the broken heart of a loving grandson.

Joy's missionary friend, Chip, was in town and he was caring for Joy and keeping her company. I was so glad for that because I couldn't devote time anywhere except to my mother and I knew Joy's desire to help me was fighting against her body's inability to do much of anything except care for itself. I thanked God for her friendship with Chip. He had accompanied her to concerts, Adam and Rita's wedding and had escorted her to the movies and to dinner during the three years she had known him. He was a special friend and with him, Joy felt like a normal woman. He bought her flowers and treated her like a lady. He ignored the appearance of her withering body and accepted her as the wonderful person that she was. His parents loved Joy and were special to her.

There were so many people in Joy's life now that I was thankful for. Most of all, I was thankful for Teri and her family for their support. I felt no longer alone — no longer fully responsible. Teri and I shared Joy's care. Debby, who was always just a phone call away and who was willing at any time to help Joy or to help me, was a great blessing. She had even been at the hospital sitting with Mother when I needed to be gone for a while. Then there was Zelda, my precious friend, who just seemed to always to know when I felt the loneliest, and she was there! People at our church were praying, upholding me during this time of pain and were on call to help with Joy, taking turns transporting her to and from her daily doctor's appointments or treatments. People from other churches in our area where Joy and I had been guest speakers, and were touched by her testimony, participated in her care and signed up to help with transportation. They were all wonderful blessings.

And last, but far from least, my compassionate and wonderful husband and our family who, even through our own crisis, anticipated Joy's needs and went out of their way to see that those needs were met while also seeing to my needs during this agonizing time in my life. God had blessed my life with flesh and blood answers to prayer as never before and I continually praised Him.

The greater the burden seemed to grow, the more grace He seemed to give. Isn't that just like God — just like my Father!

"Thank you for Chip, Debby, Judy, Helen, Debbie, Donna, Tee and Jack, Joanne and Lisa and all those women from area churches and as well, of course, from our own church, who so willingly help me get to appointments and who invite me to their homes or out to dinner and try to entertain me. I know it is not easy. Sometimes I cannot even walk up the steps to my home and yet they keep volunteering to come back. They must be tired not only of the inconvenience but it is physically tiring as well, and yet each one of them is so cheerful. They were sent by you, Lord.

Of course, Sandy, Jim and the boys and Rita and Julie and Teri and Kevin, I could not do without! Jim and Kevin must have broken backs! They have carried me up and down the stairs so often. All of them are enabling me to remain independent for all this time and I am so thankful for them. But I know it won't be too long until I will have to move. Lord, you will simply have to prepare me for that.

Sandy had to call a nursing home. Be with her, Lord. She is struggling with this!"

Chapter 37

Living Coram Deo

Joy was getting very weak again and as I had observed her for the past few days I knew that she was going to need to have another blood transfusion. Sure enough, when she called me from the doctor's office on that next morning, April 29, she had been scheduled for the transfusion that very next day. Debby called me at the hospital and made arrangements to take Joy to get the transfusion. Teri and I were so grateful for Debby. Once again, she had just volunteered to do something for Joy that enabled Teri to go to work and me not to have to worry about one more thing!

Mother was to be moved to the Hospice room in the late afternoon. Carolyn came and we bathed and changed Mother, placed her personal belongings into her overnight bag and readied her for the move. As usual Mother slept soundly through the whole ordeal, and her breathing, though labored, seemed steady.

We left the hospital to get an early dinner and upon returning we found they had already moved Mother to the Hospice room. It was a very lovely private room with a large window. Many of her nurses from the other unit came over to see us after Mother moved and told us what a privilege it had been to meet our family and to care for our mother. I felt she had received marvelous care at our local Alexandria Hospital. We thanked the Lord for those loving aides and nurses!

We arranged her room as she would have wanted it, put a stereo on her table so we could play tapes of her favorite hymns and praise choruses, and placed cherished family pictures on the shelves to remind her of our love.

We could now spend as much time with her as we wanted to without disturbing other patients and in surroundings much more like home. She would have liked the room. It was even painted in her favorite color, *pink!* As we lovingly prepared her for bed, Carolyn and I cried and hugged each other as we realized that these last days would be the most difficult we had ever faced together as a family. We didn't even need to say a word; we were both happy that we had one another!

I will always appreciate a sermon that Pastor Neil preached not too long after he came to shepherd our congregation at Faith. It was titled, *Living Coram Deo. Coram Deo* means "As before God" or "As in the presence of God."

Sometimes even as Christians we need to comprehend the fact that our lives must be lived *coram deo* because that is exactly where we are! He is ever before us — we are in His presence always. He hears, sees and knows all. Nothing is hidden from Him. Every thought and every deed is unveiled to Him.

During those final three days before the Lord took my mother home, I realized that truth as never before. I talked to Him constantly. My every heartache and every tear, I know He was aware of. I could almost feel His arms around me and I felt the touch of His hands upon my tear-stained face. I have never felt closer to Him in my whole life, and I know that I never want to be without Him — not ever! I couldn't exist without His love in my life. I want to live *coram deo* knowing that His face is always before me each and every day He gives to me on this earth. I am constantly in His presence! And to have the assurance that as I have felt His face and His presence before me on this earth, one day I will truly be in His presence and will *see* Him face to face, is the most blessed thought I can imagine!

As I think back on those heart-breaking last three days, my prayer is that my children learn the truth of that phrase *"Living Coram Deo,"* because I know once they truly comprehend it, their lives will never again be the same. Nothing they will ever face in their lives will be unbearable! It is a priceless legacy to be passed down. I pray to God that my life reflects that truth to them.

Nina was moved to a Hospice room in the hospital and the doctor told Sandy and her family that Nina would not live very much longer.

I remember a devotion that I read once when my mother was dying. It was about not being able to pray at certain times because your grief was so great but that the Spirit himself intercedes for us to the Father. The writer of the devotional said that when her sister was dying she found herself first asking the Lord to take her sister because of the pain and then she would ask the Lord not to listen to that prayer because she really didn't want her sister to die. I remember that I wrote at the bottom of that page, "Lord, that is how I feel but thank you for your love."

I know that is probably just the way Nina's family is feeling just now. "Please, Lord, put your arms around them and draw them close to you."

I am grateful for the Hospice people. I told Sandy and Teri that I want Hospice called when the time comes for me. Seems strange but I always thought God would take me long before He took Nina even though she is 92 years old! His ways are not our ways!

Chapter 38

The Homecoming Nears

During the next three days, I practically lived at the hospital. I went home for a few hours each night, and I arrived at her room by 8:00 each morning. Carolyn spent as much time as she could considering that her nursing students were in the midst of graduation.

I would bathe and change Mother and then just sit by her bed and sing to her. I held her hand as usual and prayed silently as I sang and talked to her. Andrew, Adam, Julie and Rita came by often and sat with me while talking to their Nina and telling her of their love. There were many tears mingling with hugs and kisses. Jim and Mark were there with us as time permitted with their jobs. I was always amazed how God seemed to send to me just the person I needed at the right time during those days. The pastor came in and out many times and prayed with us, as did Zelda. Others I knew were praying and I could feel those prayers.

At times Mother would open her eyes but, unlike before, it was obvious to us that she was not with us. I believe the Lord had already taken a part of her to Himself. I wondered sometimes as I watched her sleeping if she had as yet caught a glimpse of the Father as He waited for her. We still talked to her in soothing tones of love and comfort knowing that if the Lord desired, He would allow her to hear them. How I longed for that! I remembered what Pastor Neil had asked me to do and so I continued to speak to her and pray to the Lord to let her to hear my words. That gave me great peace!

April 30 I arrived at Mother's room, kissed her soft cheek and told her I loved her. She appeared to be comfortable. Christine, her Hospice nurse, had just bathed her and changed her gown and bedding.

I held her very swollen and bruised hand in mine and began to sing softly to her. As I sang, I watched the birds fluttering in the large tree just outside of her window. How Mama loved the birds and the springtime. She and I spent many hours together on our front porch and watched the little wrens as they built nests in the plants that hung there. They never seemed to be bothered by our presence there. How I wished we were there now. The world was going on outside as if nothing had changed and my world seemed to be falling apart. Why hadn't I taken time before to savor those precious times we had spent together? Why had I taken them for granted?

Thoughts of our years together flashed through my mind as I recalled the impact she had made on our family and especially on the lives of our boys. The bouquets and bouquets of "December roses" seemed to be everywhere, filling the room with their sweet fragrance. The unique family unit we shared was one of God's most cherished blessings to me and I praised Him once more for that. We had managed to combine three generations into one household for over 21 years and to do so in peace, harmony and love. I knew God was pleased, for the benefits had been realized by us all. I watched her sleep and asked the Lord to take from me what I didn't think I could do without because I knew it was best. I also knew He would say when!

Carolyn came and we spent the afternoon together. We turned Mother, bathed her still feverish body and asked that her IV which had apparently infiltrated once again, be removed and not replaced. This was a difficult decision but one that we had discussed with Hospice when we realized that to keep fluids going into a person who was dying was actually much harder on the patient than withdrawing them. We wanted her to be as comfortable as possible. Her feeding tubes had been removed days before for the same reason — it was extremely difficult for the dying patient to endure. Those decisions had been most painful, but necessary to make and we felt at peace with them.

May 1, I found Christine once again talking to Mama in sweet tones and tending to her. She had bathed and dressed her and changed her bed linens. Her hair had been brushed and she still had her pink cheeks. Her eyes were just slightly open but as I touched her face and told her I loved her, she again slipped into another world that I knew was filled with the presence of the Lord and the angels, for it was apparent that she would soon be called. Could she yet see all those who had gone on before her — the two-day-old baby girl she had lost, my grandmother, Jim's mother and father, her sisters — all waiting for her?

Joy came in against my wishes because she could barely walk and I knew she needed to save her strength. However, I also knew that it was important for her to be with me and she needed to feel useful. Joy held Mother's hand as she sat by her bedside, her eyes closed, perhaps in prayer. As I observed them I was struck by the fact that here they were the young and the old sitting together and yet both facing death — both perhaps even now reliving memories of the preciousness of life and both facing life's greatest moment for a Christian — coming face to face with Jesus. As I sat there looking at them, I praised God for the opportunity of helping them both at their journey's end!

We left Mother that evening with heavy hearts. I had never felt so lonely yet I had never felt so close to the Lord so maybe lonely wasn't the feeling — maybe it was the word *empty!* What would I do without my mother? I praised God for His nearness to me — for His faithfulness.

Chapter 39

Safely Home

It was May 2. Carolyn had called me just before I had left home to go to the hospital. The graduation for her students was over and so she would be able to be with me the biggest part of the afternoon. She had dedicated the song she had sung for the graduation, "Angels," to Mother and had challenged the newly-capped nurses to remember that in the future when they were caring for elderly patients, to remember our mother and to care for those patients in the same way they would want someone to care for their own mothers — with compassion, tenderness and most of all, with love. It was a tribute to Mother that she would have been proud of. Through her depression, Mother never thought her life had counted for much. I had spent many hours telling her what wonderful things God had done through her life — her Sunday school students who learned so many of God's truths from her, countless people who observed her life and learned from her during the many years of faithful service to the Lord in many different areas of the church, and last but not least, the lives of her children and her grandchildren touched through her godly example and her limitless and unconditional love shown to them. Lots of lives were richer because of her.

I have often been glad that we had those discussions and I was able to tell her how much she meant to me and to our boys. Most of the time it's too late when we tell our parents that we love them — most of the time they are already gone when those words are spoken. Often we just don't take the opportunity to express those feelings when it counts. Mom's depression afforded me the opportunity to do that on more than one occasion and for that I am grateful. I held on to those conversations during the rough days when my frustration level soared and during the times when neither she nor I were lovable.

Those conversations changed my life forever. I tell my children, my husband, and my friends as well, how much they mean to me. I write notes to my children that they can pull out and read when the Lord calls me home. This book is a tribute to all of my family, a legacy to the undying love I have for all of them. I hope it will serve as a challenge to them to pass that love on to their children and to their children's children. It would have first come from their grandmother, Nina!

That last day with her, May 2, 1998, when I recall it, was blessed. I spent the morning hours alone with her in our usual manner, I held her hand and continued my concert to her. Both of the boys and their wives came in during the day and kissed her and spoke to her. It would be the last time on this earth! Joy called me and she sounded very tired and lonely. I felt so sorry for her. She needed comfort and she knew that I needed it too and we could not be together. I told her to get some rest and once again I reminded her that she had to eat! She told me she was praying for me, and I knew that she was.

Carolyn came in the afternoon and together we held our mother's hands, spoke softly to her and saw that she was dry and comfortable. Mom's breathing had changed somewhat and there were other signs that her life was ending. Her face reflected peace and serenity.

Jim and Mark came in and it was decided that we would take turns going to dinner. Jim and I went to dinner with our friends Bill and Barbara Jesser who were in town. It was good to be away from the hospital for a little while and to be with Bill and Barbara once again. As you recall, they had been at our home when Mom had her first stroke. Bill and Jim were close friends from their college days at the University of Virginia. Barbara has been like a sister to me for almost forty years. She has been a prayer partner and a kindred spirit. Jim and I have cherished their friendship over those years. With them, I could be myself — no "put on a happy face," but genuine heart-to-heart conversation, mingled with laughter at just the right time. How we thank God for them.

At one point during dinner my heart was suddenly filled with a rush of heartbreaking grief even though the conversation had turned very lighthearted. Not wanting to ruin the meal for everyone, I prayed silently for the Lord's peace, dabbed my tear-filled eyes and entered into the conversation once again. Oddly enough, my sister told me that she had experienced the exact same feeling around that same time during her dinner. God was preparing us.

Carolyn had returned to the hospital but I had gone home for a few hours of rest. As I picked up our messages from the answering machine, I heard a very frantic call from Carolyn telling me that Mother's breathing was very shallow and that I should return to the hospital at once.

We arrived at the hospital to find Mother's condition very much changed from only a couple of hours earlier. Carolyn and I held her hands, kissed her cheeks and told her we loved her over and over again. Just after 11:00, Mother simply closed her still clear blue eyes, stopped breathing and slipped into the arms of Jesus, her Lord and Savior. She had waited until the four of us were there together, and then the Lord called her home. I thanked God that we were all there at that time. Jim told me later that as he stood there he had prayed that if the Lord was going to take her that night, He would do it while we were all there together. She was safely home, of that we were sure!

Nina went home to be with the Lord last night, May 2, 1998. I had just been there the day before yesterday to sit with her for a while. I knew then that it would not be long. I'm glad I made that extra effort to go to the hospital. It wasn't much but Sandy seemed to be so glad to see me. I didn't know then that it would be the last time I would see Nina on this earth.

I know just how Sandy feels today. It is all fresh in my mind even though it has been five years since my mother went to be with the Lord. I pray each night (it's the way I end my nightly prayer to Him) that the Lord will tell my mother than I love her. Sometimes it still seems as though she is only away for a little while. And yet that is true, she is only away for a little while.

I pray for Nina's family as they must go through the next several days. It will be hard on all of them and I ask God's mercy and His peace.

Chapter 40

Letting Go

Sunday, May 3, 1998 — Mother's first morning in heaven. The day was sunny and glorious; the sky brilliantly blue and crystal clear. It was as though God was reminding me of the glories of heaven, and of His infinite love and awesome power even through my broken heart.

Jim called our boys to tell them of Nina's homegoing. He said to each of them, "Your grandmother completed her journey last night and she is with the Lord."

"I liked how Dad told me about it, Mom," Andrew said when he and Julie arrived at our home that morning. "I had so much wanted her to see our baby," he said, as he sobbed in my arms. I told him I felt that God might just let her see their baby only it would be from a different location. We cried and held on to each other and I assured him that we would get through this, all of us together.

Later that evening I entered Mother's room to find Adam sitting there in the dark, rocking in her chair with tears streaming down his face. "I can smell her in this room, Mom," he said through his choking tears. "I miss her so much already." "Nina" was a very important part of his life. She was the only grandmother he had known and they were so very close.

As I held him in my arms we cried together for I knew that the tears were a sweet release that we both needed. God knew our sorrow and He understood! This wonderful young man that we had reared had tasted the bitterness of death for the first time and it was hard, but God would supply the strength.

Andrew had known his Grandma Rice for only four short years when God called her home the year Adam was born. He was the apple of her eye and he loved her dearly. I shall never forget the morning we had to tell him of her death. I held him on my lap as his father and I told him that God had taken Grandma Rice to heaven. "To do what?" he said in his sad, quivery little voice.

"Well," his father gently told him, "Jesus had a job for Grandma to do in heaven and He needed her."

"You mean like vacuuming or dusting?"

"Something like that, darling," I said as I kissed his precious face, realizing that he always observed his grandma doing something either in the house or outside in her garden!

He later said to my mother, "Grandmother, I never want you to go to heaven!" We often laughed about that when Mother would tell us through smiles that Andrew didn't want her to go to heaven!

And now here it was 24 years later and he was again having to let go of a very important part of his life. But what a privilege had been his to have had two grandmothers in his life who had both made an impression on him because of their godly examples. Andrew has made his father and me very proud of him and the person he has become especially in his walk with the Lord. We credit his grandmothers for their part in molding his life. They, too, would have been so very proud of him.

Both of my brothers made plans to come home as did Carolyn's girls and their families.

Joy came over as soon as she heard of Mom's homegoing and it was obviously most difficult for her. I knew she was reliving her own mother's death over again. She looked extremely tired and frail. I wondered just how long the Lord would tarry before he called her home too. I didn't see how she could live much longer. She ate practically nothing and her body was rapidly deteriorating before our eyes. But it was important for her to be with our family during this time; we had always been together to face times of crisis and she still needed to feel "needed."

Chapter 41

The Heaviness Of Guilt

Satan began immediately, even that day, working on my mind, filling it with guilt: "If you hadn't spent so much time working on that book of yours that you thought was so important, you would have had more time to spend with your mother. If you hadn't spent so much time with your friend, Joy, who after all is just a friend and not even your family, you would have spent more time with your mother. Shame on you, you ungrateful daughter! Call yourself a Christian? Why, you weren't even good enough to be called a friend much less a daughter. You were really no good to either one of them, you know! Sometimes you put your job ahead of taking Joy to her appointments and you shoved it off onto someone else. You could have done it all if you hadn't been so selfish. I bet both of them were really disappointed in you many times. You were not at all understanding of your mother's depression and you were impatient and sharp with her lots of times. You were even ill-tempered with her just the night before her stroke, or have you forgotten that? You slept an extra hour that morning. Remember? You were so tired, you told yourself. That is the rationale you used to justify that! Maybe if you hadn't been so self-centered and had gotten up on time, the stroke could have been managed and she would still be alive! You said that God gave you those two people to care for, and you couldn't do justice to just one of them. I'm sure that God is extremely disappointed in you. You make a lousy Christian. What a poor testimony you have been — that is, if you are honest and people know the truth. God will forget you. These years have meant nothing to Him!"

I heard those words and had those thoughts over and over again, for almost two years from the date of my mother's death. It was, I am ashamed to say, almost two years before I could finally put Satan and his guilt where they belonged, out of my life and into the hands of my Lord and Savior, Jesus Christ, that they might be crushed. It would take me those two years before I could begin to complete this book that I had promised Joy I would finish. Satan kept telling me that the book would mean nothing because I had allowed the writing of the first book to take so much time away from my mother that God wasn't even pleased with that book! Two long years I allowed Satan to strip me of joy and peace. It was during our annual women's retreat in May of 2000, that I truly turned over all that guilt to the Lord and got rid of the heavy, heavy burden I was carrying. I realized that it was not the Lord's will for me to carry that guilt. It was robbing me of doing His will for my life and it was crippling me. We had a wonderful author and retreat speaker, Joy Jacobs (see Foreword), who shared those truths with me and I made the decision to do something about it. The Lord had been ready to take that guilt from me two years before, but I didn't ever really let it go. I kept picking the guilt back up over and over again. I know the prayers of God's people had been with me for those two years and how I praise God for those prayer warriors.

During those two years, I received many phone calls and letters from people, some whom I had never met before, telling me of the impact *To Run The Race With Joy* had made on their lives. God seemed to be giving me sign after sign of His desire for me to also complete this book. Satan's lies had even tried to disguise those signs. During that retreat, God put everything into perspective for me and I called those lies what they were and my life changed. You see, Satan hits us when we are the most vulnerable and certainly I was the most vulnerable during those two years.

My dear friend, Zelda, called me the morning after my mother's homegoing and read to me the previous evening's devotional from our devotional book, *Morning and Evening* by Charles Spurgeon. Zelda had given a copy of the book to Joy and to me so we would be reading the same daily devotions. Both Joy and I loved the book so much. The selection for May 2 was titled "The Epitaph." What a blessing from God. It was about those who had died in faith and what a glorious epitaph they would have because of their faith. It was about my mother! Through tears she read to me the entire devotional and it made such an impression on me that I asked her to read it at Mother's homegoing celebration.

That book has been so precious to me many times since I started using it and especially during those last few painful weeks before Mother's death. God used it to speak to my heart and to help sustain me. Each devotional seemed to be fashioned just for my particular need at the time I needed it the most. God's provision for me was evident through that entire crisis time in my life and never more than on May 2! That devotional was indeed her epitaph!

Guilt can indeed weigh us down and make us drag. It can destroy our effectiveness as Christians. I am sorry that it took me so long to understand that. Satan has a cunning way of creeping into our lives at our weakest moments and filling our minds with his lies and his poison. The way to prevent that is through constantly keeping ourselves in His Word. I allowed my grief to keep me away from His Word because I was too busy feeling sorry for myself and too busy believing Satan's lies. I accepted them because on the surface, they seemed to be truth.

You see, God loves us unconditionally even with our faults and our failures. He doesn't ever give up on us or ever want us to feel we are useless to Him no matter what we have done. He uses our weaknesses to make us strong. Through our weakness He is the strongest. His strength is perfect when our strength is gone.

... My grace is sufficient for you, for my power is made perfect in weakness. Therefore I will boast all more gladly about my weaknesses, in insults, in hardships, in persecutions, in difficulties. For when I am weak, then I am strong.

— 2 Corinthians 12:9, 10

Chapter 42

The Epitaph

Mother's homegoing celebration was beautiful and she would have loved it. Her life was celebrated by tributes from her former Sunday school students as well as from the mother of only one of the children she had helped rear over the years. Charlie Worley, a deacon in our former church, Grace Brethren, spoke of her many years of faithful service to the Lord there in so many capacities. Her new dear friend, Zelda, from our Faith Presbyterian Church, read from Charles Spurgeon's *Morning and Evening,* "The Epitaph," May 2, and related what my mother had come to mean to her — the gentle woman who thought she had never made an impact on anyone, had indeed touched the lives of many. She was indeed loved!

Satan had also filled her mind with his lies and caused the depression from which she suffered for a number of years just as his lies had caused the guilt that had sought to consume me. How I wished I had learned the truth concerning his lies earlier so that I could have helped her through her depression. But I have managed to let that go and I have grown from my weakness and through it I have been made stronger. Mom was free from depression now and for that I praised His name!

Joy, of course, was there and had been all along. I could see her pain and I knew the last three weeks had been reminders of the painfully long death of her own mother such a short time ago. It was also a reminder of what could be in store for her perhaps in the very near future. However, we knew that our mothers were together and enjoying something beyond our wildest imaginations, and for that we both were grateful!

My brothers stayed for the week and we enjoyed being together and reminiscing about our childhood. We hadn't all been together since Mom's eightieth birthday celebration, twelve years ago. Being together did help the four of us as well as our children, with the grief process. We cried together but we also laughed; at times I felt Mom's presence with us. The healing process would take years, I knew that, and yet I could feel God beginning that healing and I praised him. Every time I looked at Julie, I was reminded of the new life within her and the promise of a baby girl to help heal our broken hearts.

When Christ was talking to His disciples about the fact that He had to leave them he said *"... Now is your time of grief, but I will see you again and you will rejoice and no one will take away your joy"* (John 16:22). We will see Mother again and then no one will take away our joy! That celebration with our loved ones who have gone before us and in the presence of the Lord face to face with Him, will not compare to any other celebration will have ever seen! Praise the Lord!

Chapter 43

Day By Day

I came to realize very quickly that this healing process was going to take a very long time. Every room in our house was filled with my mother. In her room, her clothes still smelled of her perfume. I would go to her closet and bury my face in the soft folds of the almost entirely pink wardrobe! The smell of her perfume was *"lonely."* It was a loneliness that I could not explain. Waves of it would sweep over my spirit from time to time, completely engulfing me in its depths.

I sat in Mom's room every afternoon when I came home from school and rocked in her chair and cried and prayed to God for healing. I searched for precious pictures of the two of us and held onto each and every one of them. I cherished the cards we had sent to one another with endearing words scripted therein, grateful that we were both "card savers." My first thoughts were of her each morning and my last each night.

I couldn't, however, continue to bask in my grief. I knew I had to go on with my life, painful as it was. I had a family that needed me and Joy was growing weaker by the day. She simply wouldn't eat and her weight had dropped to a mere 100 pounds! Skin and bones were all that was left of her once robust body.

Our church women's retreat was to be held the weekend of May 15-17. I had been scheduled to sing with the women's trio from our church praise band. My first impulse was to cancel but I knew Joy was looking forward to going and she wouldn't go without me. I also felt a certain obligation to my sisters in the Lord, Kathy and Debbie. I love singing with them and somehow when we sing together, my heart is so joyful.

191

I decided the Lord wanted me to go and so we went. How grateful I was that I did. The speaker, Concetta Stains, a friend of our pastor's wife, Mary Sue, was so wonderful. Her messages filled my heart, and the healing process that I so much needed was continued through her ministry. She told me later that she had prayed so fervently to the Lord to guide her to minister just the right messages that weekend and after hearing the testimony of the recent crisis in my life, she knew that God had led her to do just that. Isn't He wonderful!

Joy was so frail and so weak but her face shone with the love and light of the Lord and she, too, had needed very much to attend this retreat. It was an oasis for the two of us and it helped to heal us both in our spirits. We renewed old acquaintances there and we knew those women were still praying for both of us. I was reminded of a beautiful hymn titled "Day By Day":

> *Day by day and with each passing moment,*
> *Strength I find to meet my trials here;*
> *Trusting in my Father's wise bestowment,*
> *I've no cause for worry or for fear.*
> *He whose heart is kind beyond all measure*
> *Gives unto each day what He deems best.*
> *Lovingly, its part of pain and pleasure*
> *Mingling toil with peace and rest.*

Caroline Berg

I'm very glad that Sandy decided to go on the retreat. It was a wonderful weekend even though I know that it was hard for her to concentrate. I believe it was great timing from God.

Julie and Andrew just found out that their baby is a girl! They had invited me to go along when they went to the doctor for the ultra sound. I was excited to be asked to go and how touched I was that they did that. However, I was just too sick that day to go. How I pray that God will allow me to be able to spend a few months with their baby. Adam and Andrew seem like my brothers; actually I call them my brothers, so I will be "Aunt Joy"!

Andrew and Julie aren't telling us her name yet. That will be a surprise. I told Sandy I think they will name her Laura Brooke, Nina's mother's name, or at least part of that name. I know Sandy would be pleased if they did, but she doesn't want to think about it too much just in case I'm wrong. We really don't care what they name her, but we have fun trying to guess what it might be.

"Thank you, Lord, for letting the Rices take care of me. I love them very much!"

Chapter 44

Treatment Continues For Joy

Joy's weight continued to be a concern for the doctors. I fixed her anything and everything she could think of that she might want to eat, but she just couldn't eat it after it was prepared. She pushed her food around on her plate and tried to hide from us the fact that she had not eaten. I know she even fed some of her food to the dog because I caught her doing it! She got very good at keeping one hand at her side during meals, but we soon caught on.

The doctor gave her medicine that she called her "fat pill." It was to increase her appetite but if it did, it was very little. I used to think she didn't take the medicine at all even though she assured me that she did!

The week after the Faith retreat, Joy needed a blood transfusion because her counts were so low. She was looking forward to our beach vacation and the transfusion helped her to focus on that. Radiation was scheduled for other spots that had appeared on her spine.

The process continued, X-rays, chemotherapy, bone scans, radiation, new chemotherapy, more X-rays, radiation in new places, blood transfusions, platelets, growth factor shots. And through it all, Joy continued to want to speak anytime we were invited, sign books wherever we could and her smile was beyond belief. And vacation? She was very excited about another summer vacation at Bethany Beach, Delaware.

Teri and her family were a big part of Joy's life now and Teri had become invaluable to me with Joy's care. We decided to have a surprise birthday party for Joy in July and we had already begun to plan it.

Teri and I began to have talks about what we knew was only a matter of time — Joy couldn't continue to live alone much longer. Kevin and she had talked and decided to have Joy move in with them when, and not if, the time came. They have a house all on one floor and it made the most sense even though I knew her desire was to live with us. She had a room here and she was spending so much of her time in our home, it had become her home too. We would have to assure her that when that time came, she would still be able to spend lots of time with us. Teri agreed!

Debby and I took Joy to Washington, D.C.'s annual Race for the Cure in early June. It was a marvelous event and we even passed out lots of flyers advertising our book. Joy had a marvelous time and had chances to witness that she would not have otherwise had. I was completely exhausted by the end of the "walk" (it's hard to race uphill with a wheelchair) but we finished it and, I might add, we were not last! We took pictures and were so glad we had done that as a team!

During the months of June and July, Joy needed blood transfusions several times. We even had to take her to an oncology clinic in Lewes, Delaware, to have a transfusion while we were on vacation. The staff at the clinic were so sweet to her which made it so much easier, and we were glad that despite her having to do that, the vacation went on as usual and we had a great time. It was pretty obvious to me that it would most likely be her last summer vacation with us and I think in her heart she knew it too. We made it as normal as possible even though it was painfully clear that her body was almost spent!

We visited all of our favorite shops and restaurants. One restaurant in particular has become our favorite for an occasional family breakfast. It is the Countryside Cafe in Fenwick Island. The small, cozy restaurant has the most marvelous food. It is family owned and operated and we came to know the owners, John and Monica Tartufo, and especially two of the waitresses, Gail and Wendy. We had given them a copy of our book and they had passed it around for everyone to read. Joy loved to go there not only because of the delicious food but because she knew they genuinely cared for her. We laughed and joked with them and they treated her the way she wanted to be treated — normal!

There is a restaurant on the way to the beach in Bridgeville, Delaware, called Jimmie's Grille. We also became acquainted with several of their waitresses. One in particular, Chris Trice, became special to Joy and to me. She always asked about Joy, even when Joy wasn't with us and she, though always extremely busy in that very busy place, always found time for a hug for us and a greeting each time we were there. I gave her a copy of our book and received a marvelous letter from her telling us how very much the book had meant to her and of the recent rededication of her life to the Lord. I still keep in contact with her to this day. God has worked a miracle in that young woman's life.

I will always be grateful to those special people with whom we have come into contact. You never know how much a smile can mean to someone — what effect you could have on their life. Those wonderful people many times brought laughter and love into our lives on days that had sometimes been particularly difficult for both Joy and me. I have always tried to treat the people I meet in grocery stores, banks, shopping malls, restaurants, etc., with as much a pleasant nature as I can, because it means so much to me to be treated similarly. Also I am reminded that Hebrews 13:2 tells us, *"Do not forget to entertain strangers, for by so doing some people have entertained angels without knowing it."*

Once back from vacation, Joy decided that she wanted to be anointed. So on July 19 the elders of our church prayed, laid hands on her and she was anointed. She was prepared for God's will for her life but she also very much wanted to live. The service was wonderful and her face fairly shone with God's light.

Joy and I went to a movie together the day of her birthday, July 30. We hadn't done that for ages and we had such a fun time crying over a "chick flick." Later on that evening, we surprised Joy with a birthday party. Teri and her family and all of our family were there. She had such a great time. Tyler, her pride and joy, kissed and loved her all evening. What a buddy he had become to her. What a blessing from the Savior.

We encouraged Joy to spend the night with us. As she struggled up the stairs to bed, it was apparent that she was barely hanging on with the hustle and bustle of the evening's events, but very happy.

That was all she cared about — she knew she was loved and cared for.

And treatment continued. Her chemotherapy was constantly changed and the dreaded tests continued. The end of August, Joy's heart was only operating at 37% and the doctor started her on yet another treatment, Tamoxofin. It was very obvious that the doctors were quickly running out of options for her. They were as frustrated as she was.

We had been hearing of a new treatment for advanced breast cancer patients, called Herceptin. Some women Joy knew were getting ready to be placed on that medication and Joy wanted to see if she would be a candidate for it. Dr. Beveridge said he would check into it for her. It had serious side effects on the heart, and since her heart was having problems, it would be looked into very carefully.

We prayed for the Lord's will and the treatment. Joy, I believe, was convinced that this would be her last shot at a cure-type treatment. God was still a God of miracles but we both knew we would accept, no matter how bitter it might be.

We continued to accept speaking invitations, book-signings or whatever God had for us. Our ministry was still the focus for Joy and I believe it was what had been keeping her alive for almost two years! God's purpose for her life had been made clear to her and even though it seemed strange, she appeared to be perfectly at peace with His will no matter where it might lead. Her joy never faded, her spirit never seemed to be dark and I never heard her question her Savior. Praise to our Lord!

I can't eat! Nothing tastes good to me. The doctor gave me a "fat pill" but I don't think it's working too well!

We went on our beach vacation again. How I love that place! It's not the same because I can't do what I want to do and I feel like I can't help anymore, but I still love it there. I had to go to Lewes for treatment while we were there. The nurses were very nice and it didn't take too long. Gerrie, the Rices' neighbor at the beach, took Sandy and me. We made a fun time out of it.

I know God can heal me if it is His will. "I want to be healed — I do, Lord. Touch me just once. One touch and I know I can be healed. More than anything else, I want to live. But let me praise you through my cancer. Your will be done.

I ask to be anointed not because I think there is power in the oil, but because your Word commands it in James 5:14, 15: *'Is any one of you sick? He should call the elders of the church to pray over him and anoint him with oil in the name of the Lord. And the prayer offered in faith will make the sick person well; the Lord will raise him up. If he has sinned, he will be forgiven.'* I was anointed once before. I feel that each day you give me is a healing of sorts for I have been given another day to serve you. I just celebrated another birthday. With this new treatment that I have been found to be a candidate for, maybe this is my healing — don't know. ˉ

Your will be done. I trust you, Lord."

Chapter 45

Mother's Gift And God's Glory

We were anxiously awaiting the birth of our granddaughter and news from Joy's doctor concerning her shot at the new treatment. We were scheduled to speak at another women's retreat, at a Life With Cancer group at Fairfax Hospital, and I was to speak at the Northern Virginia Christian Writers' Association meeting. The months of September and October were quickly filling. Life was going on but my heart was still hurting with an indescribable hurt. I couldn't seem to get past it a little bit, much less beyond it!

Then one day my sister called me and said, "Sandy, I found something today in that file cabinet that belonged to Mother and I want to read it to you. You know, I went through and cleaned out that file cabinet three times and I can't believe I did not see this before. It must have been placed there for us at this particular time and when I read it to you I want you to accept this as a gift from Mom and let us go on with our lives. She wants us to do that. Are you listening to me?"

"Yes," I answered with anticipation filling my troubled heart.

She then read to me a poem written anonymously titled "Safely Home."

Safely Home

I am home in Heaven, dear ones;
All's so happy, all's so bright!
There's perfect joy and beauty
In this everlasting light.

All the pain and grief are over,
Every restless tossing passed;
I am now at peace forever,
Safely home in Heaven at last.
Did you wonder I so calmly
Trod the Valley of the Shade?
Oh! but Jesus' love illumined
Every dark and fearful glade.
And He came Himself to meet me
In that way so hard to tread;
And with Jesus' arm to lean on,
Could I have one doubt or dread?
Then you must not grieve so sorely,
For I love you dearly still;
Try to look beyond earth's shadows,
Pray to trust our Father's will.
There is work still waiting for you.
So you must not idle stand;
Do your work while life remaineth —
You shall rest in Jesus' land.
When that work is all complete,
He will gently call you home;
Oh, the rapture of the meeting!
Oh, the joy to see you come!

It seemed to be words directly from our Mother! She had experienced so many "restless tossings" and now they were truly passed. The Lord himself was there to meet her. She and I had discussed so many times her fears, and there it was "and with Jesus' arm to lean on could I have one doubt or dread?" Mother had once told one of her companions she didn't feel afraid to die, but she knew from what I had told her, that I would grieve so if she left. And there it was, "Then you must not grieve so sorely, for I love

202

you dearly still." And then quite clearly she wanted us to continue here on this earth doing God's work until He called us home, "Do your work while life remaineth."

I cannot tell you what that "gift" meant to me and to this day I cherish that poem. I have it almost memorized. And to think that it was placed there in that cabinet, overlooked three times, until the very time we needed it the most. Had it been found before that time, it may have been tossed away for it was yellowed with age and crumpled up. Jim's mother had passed it on to my mother years before and it was placed there to be found at just at the right time. God's timing was so very perfect. My heart was filled with wonderful peace and the presence of my mother. Carolyn and I accepted that as Mother's gift for us and for all those who grieved for her. I made copies of the poem and gave them as gifts to our children and grandchildren. It has become a most loved "gift." Each time I feel the waves of grief, I have just to remember a line of that poem and it brings great comfort to me.

God showed to me His awesome power and glory once more the next week when Jim and I made a trip to the cemetery. We had received a call from the cemetery telling us that Mother's name-plate had been installed, and we needed to inspect it for accuracy.

The day was bright and glorious as we left for the cemetery only a very short distance from our house. My heart again felt heavy for I hadn't visited the cemetery since Mother's funeral. We parked the car and walked the few short yards to the grave site. As I stood there looking at the nameplate through a veil of tears, I realized anew that her death was indeed real; she was gone and I would not see her again on this earth. I knew that but this made it so — so — final!

We had been there but a few seconds when the sky grew very dark almost like night, and the wind began to blow with such force that the straw that had been laid down to protect the newly sewn grass seed, was picked up and thrown at us with all the strength of a tornado. The flying straw and other debris stung our faces and forced us to run towards the car shielding our eyes.

Once inside the car we sat for a few minutes and watched the whirlwind display outside. As we drove from the cemetery I looked at Jim and told him through my tears that is was as if God were telling me that I did not need to stand and grieve at that grave for my mother, for she was not there — she was with Him and safe — Safely Home!

On the way down our street, only about five minutes later, the sun appeared once again, and the darkness dissolved into glorious brilliant azure blue skies. God had shown me once again through His marvelous power that He was in control and that I need not fear. With Mother's precious gift to me and God's show of power, might and glory, what more could I possibly need?

Chapter 46

God's Precious Gift

Joy and I spoke at a Life With Cancer group at Fairfax Hospital on October 19. It was a small group, but I knew from the questions we were asked that it was just the group God Himself had assembled. Teri, Joy and I were excited at the opportunity we had been given, and we sold quite a few books.

Joy was to have her first Herceptin treatment the next day and our baby was to be born very soon! Andrew had called his father while we were at our meeting and told him that the doctor had decided to induce labor on Julie and the baby would probably be born either later that night or the next morning. Needless to say, we were elated. I could hardly sleep!

Joy had spent the night at our house and Teri was going to pick us up the next morning. We were going to be with her for the six hours she was scheduled to take the Herceptin. Because it was relatively new, and Joy's heart was certainly not operating at full capacity, there was a chance she could have a heart attack with the first dose! She was nervous, but at the same time this treatment was her last chance and she wanted to take it!

Andrew called us very early the morning of October 20 and said that it was decided to perform a Caesarean section on Julie. He assured us that Julie and the baby were just fine but it had been a difficult night. Andrew told us that if we arrived at the hospital around 8:00, the baby would be born and ready for company and Julie would probably be ready to go to her room. Jim and I dressed quickly and after seeing that Joy was dressed and waiting for Teri, we kissed her and left for the hospital. We assured her that Jim and

I would be with them to have prayer before she was to have the Herceptin. It was scheduled to begin at 9:00.

Andrew looked exhausted when he met us just outside the delivery room but I have never seen such a glow on his face! At 8:30 he came out wheeling the most beautiful baby girl I had ever seen in my whole life. "Let me introduce you to your granddaughter, Amanda Brooke Rice," he proudly said!

I cannot even relate to you my feelings and emotions at that precious moment. I was completely overcome with so much joy in my heart that it was indescribable! The three of us hugged and cried. It was an awesome feeling to be looking at our son's baby! And the name: Amanda Brooke! My mother's mother's name was Laura Brooke. She was always called, "Brooke." My mother would have been thrilled beyond words to have known that the baby's name was to be Amanda Brooke. I believe God told her and that He allowed her to see her precious great granddaughter that day, for the room seemed to be filled with the light of heaven itself as I gazed into the face of that little angel!

This baby, God's blessed gift to our family, would be loved and cherished by our family always. She was to be the healing for our hearts, for the healing process had begun months ago as we anticipated this day.

Jim and I left the hospital that morning and hurried across the street to have prayer with Joy before her treatment was to begin. As we prayed for Joy and held her hands, I knew that the Father was faithful — always faithful. Joy had tears in her eyes as we told her all about the baby, and promised we would take her to see Miss Amanda Brooke Rice that very evening!

Joy had prayed for God to allow her a little time to spend with this precious baby, and He was going to give her that desire of her heart. Something else to focus on right now was what she needed.

Joy's treatment went very well, and the doctors seemed pleased. Adam and I went back and forth between the hospital and the doctor's office showing Joy videos of the baby and visiting with Julie, Andrew, and Amanda. It made the long day much better for Joy as well as for the rest of us. Joy had a look of radiance on her face as she anticipated going home and then to the hospital to see Amanda.

When I watched Joy's face as she held Amanda in her arms that evening, I thanked God for his amazing grace. All I could think of was God is so Good — God is so Good. His precious gift was filling something in our hearts that only she could and God had provided her just in time — just in time for us all!

Herceptin began today and it went pretty well except I was so tired at the end. Amanda Brooke Rice was born this morning. She is beautiful. I got to hold her tonight. "Thank you, Lord, for allowing me to see her. Your will be done, now."

Chapter 47

A Dream Fulfilled

Debby and I had discussed what we would like to do for Joy — something that she would really like to do before the Lord took her home. We looked into an organization out of California called the Dream Foundation, which is designed to fulfill special wishes for adults with terminal illnesses.

You see, Joy had no desire to travel worldwide (nor could she) or to meet famous people simply because they were famous. But her real desire was to meet celebrities whose lives she could perhaps touch for the Lord, and because of their celebrity status, if they were led by Him, could touch multitudes!

Early in September, she had been flown to New York (arranged by her friend Katie Couric) where she met Rosie O'Donnell. She was able to hand our book personally to Rosie and to say a few words to her. Rosie did promise Joy she would read the book and we trust God that she will. That meeting was really fulfilling for Joy but, above all, I knew Joy's heart's desire would be to meet Oprah Winfrey!

"Just think what Oprah could do if she heard our story and was moved by what God has done," Joy once said to me as we watched *The Oprah Show* one afternoon. "She has so much influence through her large audiences! Our story told by her would be a dynamite testimony!"

So I called the Dream Foundation and found out what we had to do in order to get her to Chicago and lunch with Oprah Winfrey. I had in the past written many letters to Oprah and entered several of her contests trying to get Joy onto her show because I thought she would make a terrific guest in light of her marvelous reaction to her cancer, but I had gotten no response from Oprah's staff. We received the forms from the Dream Foundation, filled out our part and then Teri and I took the form to Dr. Beveridge for his signature.

"You are off the charts you know," he told her as he was looking over the form. "I wouldn't have given you nearly this much time according to all of our statistics. You are a marvel! I'm going to list your life expectancy at five months only so your name will go to the top of the list, young lady, because I long ago gave up predicting your situation. I'll do this for you only if you promise to mention my name to Oprah!" he said, with a twinkle in his eye.

"I will definitely tell her you are the best doctor in the world," Joy answered, as he laughed and continued his routine examination.

Teri and I were glad for the laughter because as we faced each other we knew that we were both thinking the same thing; he had put "five months" because that was most likely a very good "guess." It was the first time we had gotten any prognosis at all from anyone. Perhaps it had been the best way after all — not knowing — for we were to soon find out that he was right almost down to the day! The cancer had just about completed its deadly task. There was simply no part of her body that had not been affected by it, and we were all painfully aware of that. However, one had only to reflect on her name, Joy, see her face still radiant with the love of Jesus Christ, and watch her struggling with every ounce of energy she still had left, to remember that cancer was powerless to penetrate her heart and her soul! She had won the victory and no one or nothing could take that from her! That thought would serve to sustain us throughout the coming days, the very few days, that were left!

I mailed the forms back to California and anxiously awaited an answer. On the way back from the mailbox, my mind drifted back to that lazy afternoon so many months ago just after we received our first copies of the book. We were plopped down on my bed laughing as we reminisced and giggled at the prospect of meeting Oprah, having her tell us how much she liked our book and inviting us on her show!! And now it appeared as if we might do just that — well, we were at least going to meet her for lunch! Our main prayer was that we could give her our book in person, have a chance to share our faith, and pray that the Lord might lead her to read our book, and in its pages she might see that we had found the truth to real joy through Jesus Christ.

The Dream Foundation answered our letter pretty quickly but a call from them shortly thereafter revealed that they were unable to arrange a luncheon with Oprah; however, we were definitely assured of attending a taping of one of her shows. Joy and I would fly to Chicago, all expenses paid, and receive hotel accommodations and tickets to the taping. The dates were set for November 16-20. We could have had tickets for the theater and other sightseeing and television shows, but we really didn't want to be away from home that many days and I was beginning to be fearful of being away from Joy's doctors for too long. Two days there would be plenty. We arranged to go from November 16-18. Joy could hardly wait!

At the end of September, the Dream Foundation called us and offered Joy and me the opportunity to go to the French Riviera! A wealthy couple had booked the trip and then had to cancel so they donated their entire trip — one week with all expenses paid — to the Dream Foundation! Shannon, our contact at the Dream Foundation, wanted to offer the trip to Joy and me in addition to our trip to Chicago! We were flabbergasted! Of course it was out of the question because first of all we had no passports and secondly, we didn't think Joy could get permission from her doctors to go out of the country. Even if we had received the okay from the doctor, I would have been scared to death to take her that far! I was getting more and more frightened to take her even a few miles away from home! However, we told everyone about our chance and we dreamed about it anyway!

Joy called her best friend from college, Brenda Patterson, who teaches in Chicago, and told her about our pending trip. We made plans to visit with her and it was our hope to get her in to see Oprah, too, if we could. Joy was getting more and more excited. The color was back in her cheeks and she seemed to be doing pretty well except for the fact that she was tired all the time. I began to wonder whether or not going that far was a good idea.

We asked the Dream Foundation to arrange for a wheelchair at the airport and the hotel, and they called us to say that it was done! They were super to work with and anxious to do whatever they could in order to fulfill Joy's dream. Joy could now go nowhere without the wheelchair! She did fairly well with her walker in her condo and for short jaunts, but the wheelchair had become a necessity. She really didn't fight it too much because she knew it was that or she could not go anywhere at all!

It was during this planning period for our trip that Debby and her husband and family moved to Ohio. Scott had been offered a good job there and had accepted the opportunity. It was heartbreaking for us all to tell them goodbye. How I would miss Debby and Scott and the kids. They had become such an important part of our family and Debby had been such a support to Joy and to our "team." Whatever would I do without her? She would be close to our Sherry who also lives in Ohio, and I was glad for that; but what would I do?

Through many tears and with many lengthy phone calls and visits leading up to the day they left, we said our goodbyes to them. Even though I knew they had sought God's will for their move, I was a little angry with God. I had been dependent upon Debby and now she would be gone. I knew God would continue to supply our needs but no one could take Debby's place — no one! I promised her that I would tell her every little detail of our trip to Chicago, for she and I had planned it together.

Almost immediately, Teri volunteered to take Debby's place on our team by agreeing to attend retreats, book-signings and other engagements with us. I thanked God for her willingness. God had answered prayer assuring us once again that He had everything under control. As I informed Debby of Teri's willingness to help, I knew she had had her prayers answered too, for she knew we would need someone to help us, and she felt badly about not being able to do it anymore.

Joy and I left for Chicago early on November 16. Jim drove us to the airport, helped us with our luggage and saw that our wheelchair was available. I wished he had been going with us — I hated to feel so responsible for Joy all by myself. I knew that I would feel much better once we met up with Brenda.

Joy did very well on our flight. I still find flying very stressful and I am always glad when we land. The neatest thing about this particular flight was that we flew "first class"! There had been a mixup in our flights. As a result, the aisle seats that we had requested because of Joy's need to have her left leg to the outside of the seat, were not available for us. Joy talked to the airlines and convinced them to upgrade our seats! What a difference!! First class is definitely the way to go, we decided. We pretended to be important passengers as we received "celebrity" treatment. We had a ball acting our usual silly selves. I don't think the flight attendant had ever encountered such crazy passengers but we had her laughing, too!

We met with Brenda that evening. I could tell by the tears in her eyes when she first saw Joy that she was fearful that this would be the last time she would see her here on this earth. It was obvious that she was shocked by Joy's frail appearance. We went to dinner and talked Brenda into spending the night with us in our room. We ordered a cot and since we had spoken to her earlier in the day, Brenda had brought her clothes just in case we were able to arrange a place for her to bunk with us.

What a great time we had, the three of us together. We talked until very late. Joy, most excited about the next day's trip to meet Oprah, slept very little and therefore neither did I! She was awake at 4:00! We talked quietly when we couldn't sleep, trying not to awaken Brenda; however, by 6:00 we were all awake so we decided we might as well get dressed and get going!

We were able to get Brenda into the studio with us. We watched a taping of the first birthday party of the McCaughey septuplets. It was a cute show with all the babies, and for a first-time grandmother, it made me miss my Mandy all the more.

After the taping, Oprah came out on stage and talked to the audience. She asked if a Joy Seale was in the audience and when Joy loudly said, "Yes," she asked her to come down on stage. Of course we had to get help with her wheelchair and I was asked to come with her. I could almost hear Joy's heartbeat as we got to the platform.

Oprah hugged us both and introduced Joy and me to the audience. She told Joy that Katie Couric had told her all about Joy and her courageous fight with cancer and about Joy's desire to meet her. She thanked me for being such a wonderful friend to Joy as she told her audience that I had become Joy's primary caregiver and what an important role that was. She then asked Joy to tell the audience a bit about herself and our book. Joy asked Oprah if she had received the book we had sent to her by the Dream Foundation, and she assured Joy that she had it.

For the next five or ten minutes Joy addressed the audience with her testimony of the Lord's grace and how He was using her life through her cancer. She told them that her desire was that each of them realize that it wasn't the amount of time you were given on this earth that counted but what you did with the time you had and that her desire was to glorify God in the time she had left. It was a powerful testimony and you could feel the spirit of God in that place. Several people spoke to her afterwards about her testimony.

Oprah presented to Joy a huge basket filled with books, food, clothing, lotions and soaps. She said she had filled it with some of her favorite things because she wanted Joy to have the things that she, too, loved. We had to buy an extra suitcase just to carry those items home! It was a very exciting time for Joy but she was the most joyful to again be able to give her testimony.

I don't know whether or not that meeting made any life-changing impression on Oprah. That is not up to us — we only sow the seed. We don't know whether or not she read our book — that also is up to God. I do know that Joy fulfilled her dream and God will not return it void! We know that we did all that we could to sow that seed in the short time we were given, and we know that God will honor that.

We left Chicago with tears in our eyes as we said goodbye to Brenda, but with joy in our hearts having fulfilled a dream for Joy — to use one more opportunity to witness for her Lord, and this time to one of the most powerful women in the country!

May His will be accomplished! *"... so is my word that goes out from my mouth: It will not return to me empty, but will accomplish what I desire and achieve the purpose for which I sent it"* (Isaiah 55:11).

It was a dream come true to meet Oprah Winfrey. Not just because she is famous but because I got a chance to witness to her and the audience. I know God will honor that and my prayer is that she will read our book and her heart will be touched.

We had a great time, Sandy, Brenda and I. I will miss times like that! Brenda has been special to me for many years. I love her and wish she lived closer to us. She cried when we told her goodbye. I will miss her and our friendship, and I thank God that she was in my life.

Sandy and I enjoyed our trip home on the airplane. We have had such a good time over these last few days. My mind was filled with fond memories as I looked over at her and thought how hard it will be when I have to leave her — when the Lord takes me home. Then I thought of Teri and how hard it will be on her once the Lord takes me, just when we have become close again. And Ty! I wish I could live to see him grow up and become a man but I know that is not possible. I hope he remembers me and how much I loved him. And Trisha, Lord! She is a really good kid. I wish the best for her. My prayer is that Teri, Kevin, Tyler and Trisha come to know the Lord in a very real way. Teri knows the truth, she has just gotten a little lost. My one desire is for all of them to get back to church like a family and to love the Lord!

Jim met Sandy and me at the airport and took us to dinner at a very fancy restaurant before they drove me home. What a nice surprise! It felt good with all three of us together again. They took me home and helped me into my condo and then they left to go see baby Amanda. They are so good to me and I praise God for them.

Chapter 48

We Face The Truth — Together

Once back from Chicago, we had to make our holiday plans. I had really thought that Christmas, 1998, would have been Joy's last here on earth, but God had spared her for yet another one and I hoped we could make it special because she and I both knew time was precious.

The stairs continued to be such a struggle for her. Even though she weighed just under 100 pounds, it was also becoming difficult for us to carry her. Andrew and Adam did most of her grocery shopping and they took turns getting her mail for her and carrying out the trash.

When one of Joy's neighbors, Donna, inquired as to what she might do in order to help Joy, I asked if she might be able to get the mail for Joy since she had to stop to get hers anyway. She graciously offered to do that. After persuading Joy that people wanted to help and didn't know what to do, she agreed, albeit reluctantly.

So many of her neighbors and friends very much wanted to be able to do something. I finally made Joy realize that she needed to accept help when it was offered because these friends were sent by God to minister to her. Donna became such a blessing to Joy as did her downstairs neighbors, the Bouldens, Tee and Jack. They are a marvelous Christian couple and were so helpful to Joy during the last few months she was able to stay in her condo. Joy and I loved them and I thank God for them. People had been placed by God into Joy's life in remarkable ways! Once she realized that, she began willingly to accept any help that was offered. Their help freed up our family and Teri's family as well, to be able to do the things for her that none of them could. It was a tremendous help to

217

us and we thanked God for all who were such a blessing to her and to us during those last few months.

Right before Christmas, Joy and I talked seriously for the first time about her death. "I know that I am dying and that I don't have much time left," she said to me matter-of-factly one day!

"Why do you say that?" I asked, as I looked her squarely in the face.

"I just feel it in my body. I am very tired and I have nothing left to fight with! You know it's true. I know you do! I'm not afraid. Really I'm not. But I wish I had longer. I honestly wish I had longer."

With that, I didn't know what to say, and so I said nothing. What was there to say? I knew it was true. All the jokes and snappy comebacks seemed so inappropriate just then. No laughter this time, just a quiet acceptance of the inevitable. She was dying and very soon! We exchanged glances that said volumes without words. We would see it through until the end — together!!

"Christmas is near and I thank you, Lord, for yet another one." My devotion for today, December 18, is taken from Joel 2:13: *"Rend your heart and not your garments. Return to the Lord your God, for he is gracious and compassionate, slow to anger and abounding in love, and he relents from sending calamity."* It tells me that I have to rend my heart and the only way to do that is to take my heart to Calvary and to let the Lord himself rend it as only He can, to make it what He wants it to be. I want my life every day to be real and not phony. I want my heart to be soft and ready to be used by Him. "Lord, help me to take my heart to Calvary each new day to be made the way you want it to be."

I asked the Lord to be with Sandy at this time — the first Christmas without her mom. I can relate to that very well because I have been there. But God has already made it different for her by sending Amanda. She may not see it all clearly yet, but I know Amanda is going to make a difference, not only in this Christmas, but in the months to come.

My foot hurts so badly today, and it stays so cold. Never has cold been so *cold.* The pain is terrible and sometimes I'm afraid the doctor will have to cut my foot off. I pray that doesn't happen! I want to keep my legs! I cry with pain sometimes, but at least it comes and goes and is not constant.

Jim picked me up to go to their house for dinner. I can eat hardly at all so Jim stopped by and bought me a taco because he knows I like them. He treats me special in a lot of different ways. He is so thoughtful and I love him very much. It was nice to be with my "family" again.

Sandy and Jim took me home and carried me up the stairs. I hope Jim doesn't break his back — I know it is hard on both of them. They said we would get a Christmas tree tomorrow and I will be there for the decorating. It will be fun. I hope my leg doesn't hurt tomorrow. I am going to take a bath now and maybe the warm water will help my foot.

"I thank you, Lord, for another day! And, thank you for my wonderful family, and for the family of God, and my neighbors. I know you will call me home soon. I will accept your will."

Chapter 49

Home For Christmas

I took a trip to the cemetery on the morning of December 23 to place some holly and pine at Mother's grave site. She loved holly so much. Her favorite tree in our yard was the holly tree. She loved the dark red berries and the beautiful lush green leaves it displayed — especially at Christmas time. The tree was always full of singing birds.

The air was very cold and the bitter wind stung my face as I walked from my car to the site. The marble, too, felt very cold as I touched it to remove the vase, but I knew that the spirit of the one whose earthly body was placed there was warm and more alive than ever before.

I arranged the foliage after removing the lovely pink silk spring flowers that Adam and I had placed there months ago. Fragments of two once fresh rose buds were also in the vase. Their petals had only recently dried and fallen off, for they were strewn about the base of her crypt. Someone who had loved her had placed them there. Though I didn't know who had honored her so, it gave me great joy to know she had been remembered.

I stood there for a few moments with hot tears streaming down my bitter cold cheeks. I longed to kiss her just once more. The hurt surfaced and the wound in my heart felt fresh again. I kissed my finger and pressed it hard into her nameplate and hurried off to the warmth of my car.

I talked to the Lord all the way home as Christmas carols played softly on the radio. As He spoke to my heart I realized that Mother was experiencing the greatest Christmas of her whole life this year, for she was with her Lord. She was remembering only the love she had on this earth, not the pain or sorrow of life, but the love — the love we shared with her.

As the snowflakes fell for most of the day, and the carols played throughout the house, I no longer pictured the cemetery as cold and lonely, but as a place where, when I go, I can reflect on a life that was more alive on the day we placed it there, than it ever was before. For us, as saints, the last date on that piece of stone or bronze is really the first day of our eternal life. And for my mother, May 2, 1998, was that day. This year she was truly home for Christmas!

And what would next Christmas bring? Would I find myself in that very same cemetery standing at Joy's grave site? Would I remember what I had learned this day? What would the last date on her plate of bronze reflect? How long would it be from this date to that one? I didn't know the answer to any of those questions but I knew who did and I knew that He would sustain me from now until that time and even forevermore, until my own earthly body would be placed at that same cemetery and I, too, would be more alive then than ever before, and rejoicing with both Joy, my dearest friend, and my precious mother.

Chapter 50

A Cherished Christmas

Christmas Eve breakfast, a new tradition, was wonderful — all of us together including Joy, of course. And now a new little gift, especially from the Father, Amanda Brooke!

What a blessing we had received. Her very presence filled the room with love! I was glad that Joy was getting to spend this Christmas with Amanda, too. She was a reminder that God is faithful and that life is precious. She had already began a healing in our hearts after the death of Mother and she would continue to help heal our hearts in the months to come. She was also preparing us for another void in our lives that would soon become apparent to us all.

Joy spent Christmas Eve night with Teri and her family. She was looking forward to seeing Tyler on Christmas morning and he was so happy that she would be there. She came back to our house Christmas afternoon and spent the rest of the day with us. We had Jim's brother and sister-in-law, Martin and Joanne, and their extended family there, and with our boys and their families, including our little Missy Mandy, it was a wonderful day, but not quiet! It was family! Joy had enjoyed a wonderful Christmas and it was evident as her eyes, though tired, sparkled in the reflection of the Christmas tree lights!

Joy had added her own "special" tree ornament to our tree, as you recall was her custom. This year's selection wasn't nearly as, shall we say, "flamboyant" as usual! We laughed as we pointed out the ornaments of past years, including the *Liberty Bell* she had purchased on a previous Christmas. Each ornament on our tree has special meaning to our family — the ones the boys made in

223

school with their colored macaroni frames and school pictures pasted inside; the lace and cinnamon ornaments Mom and I had made together; the ones given to us by special friends; those purchased on vacations; the red heart carefully scripted with the name "Nina" given to her by a dear neighbor; our latest ornament adorned with a picture of our littlest angel, Amanda; and, of course, those ornaments selected by Joy as her special additions. These are the things that help to make up "family" — special traditions and memories.

I will miss these times with Joy as I miss them with my mother — the laughter and the special things we shared. However, I remembered those "roses in December" and I realized that we had gathered yet another bouquet for cold and perhaps lonely Decembers to come. So as everyone went home and I had gathered up the last "rose" for the bouquet, I snuggled into bed beside my husband and, feeling his warm embrace, I knew that I was a very blessed woman. I praised the Father for His Son — the most blessed gift of all time!

New Year's Eve came and went with no particular fanfare. We spent it quietly with Joy, Andrew, Julie and our little darling, Mandy. I recalled last New Year's Eve when Joy, Jim and I had part of our Bible study class in our home for the evening. We played musical charades and Mom and I were a team. She would whisper the song in my ear and I would act it out. We had such a good time and such laughs. Had I known it was to have been her last New Year's Eve with us I would have held onto it a little tighter — just a little tighter. I seemed to be holding onto this one as tightly as I could but I knew I had to let it go.

Another year was here! The past year had been a painful year for me and I knew 1999 would be painful also. But I also knew that God had gone before me and He would lead us all through whatever was before us. His Word tells us in John 17:17 that *"Thy Word is truth."* I knew that the Word of God would never lead us contrary to the will of God and that He would never lead us where His grace could not keep us. We believe as did David in Psalm 61:3, 4 that He is a strong tower against the foe and we can take refuge in the shelter of His wings. I knew that those wings were just a prayer away and that brought great comfort to my weary-worn body!

I woke up on Christmas morning at Teri's house. I thanked God for sending His son, Jesus Christ, to the world and for giving me eternal life. I thanked Him for giving Sandy and her family to me and for Teri and Kevin and their family. I am very blessed.

We had fun yesterday morning at the Rices. Jim fixed a great breakfast and the kids came with little Brooke. (I like to call her "Brooke." That is her middle name.) We always have a good time together. They care for me and always worry and fuss over me just like I was their own. I love them so much.

I had a great time with Teri, Kevin, Tyler and Tricia this morning. I gave Teri a cross that I had bought when she went shopping with me. She thought I bought it for Tricia. Boy, was she surprised! I wrote her a letter with it and she cried. We both cried together and ended the morning with tight hugs. I will miss them and the memories we have had together. I wish I could see the kids grow up. I want them to learn to love the Lord as I do and to serve Him as a family. That is my prayer for them always. I love them all so very much. I'm thankful that they love me, too.

Christmas day with the Rices has been a tradition for several years now. They **always** include me. Teri took me to their house and we had our present opening time. Jim's brother and his family were over for dinner. I love them, too. Jim's sister-in-law, Joanne, and her daughter, Lisa, have been so sweet to me. They have taken me to doctor's appointments many times. I know it has been hard sometimes for them to do that. Lisa has a baby and Joanne herself has breast cancer. But they never seem to mind. I pray for Joanne all the time.

Sandy's sister, Carolyn, and her family have been very supportive to me also. I thank God for them and love them. It's like the Rices' whole family just adopted me! I am blessed.

Rita and Adam left Christmas night to drive down to see Rita's parents. I hope they drive safely. I worry about them. Rita's mother and father will be happy to see them. We really love Bettie and

Louis. Rita's family prays for me all the time. I get e-mails from Rita's sister, Maria, telling me that. Many people pray for me. I thank the Lord for them all.

"I have had a very wonderful Christmas, Lord, but I am very tired and very cold. Thank you again, Lord, for giving me eternal life by dying for me."

Chapter 51

Total Dependence - The Inevitable

Joy experienced her first panic attack on January 6. Her friend, Chip, had taken her for a Taxol treatment and she had suffered a panic attack at the hospital. The nurses had calmed her down and Chip had driven her home. Teri was at Joy's condo to spend the night with her and after hearing of the panic attack she became frightened. She finally got hold of me when I got home from school. She was almost hysterical. I suggested that they get Joy oxygen because it might make her feel better. She kept thinking she couldn't breathe. Chip came over to our house where I had secured a tank of oxygen from my neighbor who just happens to use oxygen from time to time and had an extra tank. Chip took it to Joy but Teri never had to set it up.

It was a frightening experience for us all and I realized that it was just the beginning of frightening experiences. I needed to be strong not just for Joy but for Teri as well. It was to be a long road.

"I was really scared that I was going to die right there in the hospital," Joy confided to me the next day. "I wasn't afraid to die, but I didn't want to die without you around."

"I'm so sorry you had to go through that and I'm sorry that I wasn't there for you. But you know you are never alone. The Lord is always there." I felt guilty not having been there and I didn't quite know what to say to her. I couldn't go with her to every appointment and she was aware of that and had accepted it. Her appointments were becoming almost a daily thing and I had to work. Still, I knew what she really wanted was for me to be there.

"I know you can't always be there, Sandbox, I really do. Don't feel bad. I didn't mean to make you feel sad. Just promise me that you will be with me when things get really bad. I don't want to be in a place where I don't know anyone when the end comes. Okay?"

"I promise you won't be with people you don't know. We will be with you. Count on it." And having made that pact we hugged as we shed a few tears and I prayed that I could live up to that promise.

Joy's heart was a concern to her doctor. She continued to be so very short of breath. She could not walk and talk at the same time. I was worried about the effect the Herceptin was having on her heart and lungs. Teri took her to the doctor and they scheduled her for a heart test on January 8. Teri planned to take her. The doctor wanted the results of the test faxed to him as soon as possible after the test. Teri and I knew that he was very worried. We were to take her to the doctor on January 9.

It snowed on Thursday night and so Joy spent the night at our house. School was canceled for the next day and I was glad because I would be able to accompany Joy to the doctor. We got up and ate a leisurely breakfast with Adam who had brought donuts over (one of Joy's favorites). Teri picked us up at noon and we went together to see the doctor.

Just as I had suspected, the Herceptin was adversely affecting her heart and the treatments had to be stopped. She was to have no medication at all for two weeks and he wanted to call Hospice into her case. He assured her that she could be taken out of the Hospice program if she improved — Teri and I knew that she would not be taken out of Hospice. I think Joy knew that too. Teri and I together told Dr. Beveridge that we wanted to have in-home Hospice.

The doctor advised that Joy move out of her condo for at least two weeks. Because she would not be having any treatment and because her heart was so weakened, she could not be alone. That was a difficult pill for her to swallow. She knew that once she moved, she would not be going home again. Teri and I knew that this was a final move for her and we had a difficult time holding back the tears. We tried to lighten up the conversation on the way home, but we all felt the same thing — a sense we were losing each other and yet we had to hold together. We had to fight to hold together, but God would be our strength.

Teri and Kevin had been making plans for weeks to have her move in with them. We had discussed it at length and as hard a decision as it was for me, I had to accept it. Teri and Kevin had their living quarters on one level. She could have a bedroom, bath, and access to the living room and kitchen, all on one floor. It would be the best solution. I felt guilty at not being able to have her stay in our home and yet it would have been foolish to try. She would always have felt guilty because I would have to go up and down the stairs endlessly, and she would feel far away from the family much of the time because the kitchen and family room are downstairs. There is no full bath on our first floor — it wasn't practical at all. I told Teri that our family would help get her house ready for Joy's move, assist in the move and that she could count on us to continue as a team to help them to care for Joy. I realized that Teri needed to do this for Joy as well as for herself. They had always relied on each other like sisters when they were growing up, and now they needed each other as they never had before. And so on January 10, 1999, we moved Joy into Teri and Kevin's house. I could tell by Joy's face when we got her settled in that she knew this was to be permanent. It almost broke my heart.

Dr. Beveridge had also told us that Joy needed to have pretty much full time care for those two weeks. In order for Teri and me to save our leave so we could use it further down the road, I arranged for women from our church and other churches in the area, who had wanted to help with Joy's care, to take shifts during the day to stay with Joy. They were all eager to help and I had no trouble at all finding volunteers. The problem was JOY!

"I don't need babysitters, Sandbox!" she said almost in tears as she called me at work two days later. "I know they want to help but I feel like I have to entertain them and I don't feel like it. Do you understand? I can stay by myself. I don't need anyone 24 hours a day. I have the phone and Kevin comes in and out of the house all day long. Please!" she begged.

Helen, the chairman of our Diaconate at church, had worked very hard to get volunteers signed up and coordinated with the list I had made of others who wanted to help. I was physically as well as emotionally exhausted with that, coupled with the move. I didn't need Joy's stubbornness to boot — not now! I told Joy I would consult with Teri and Hospice and try to lessen the help if I could.

"Just go with it for a couple of days and I'll see what I can do. Okay? You have to give me time to work this out. So be nice to the ladies, little girl, and I'll get back to you," I said, with sarcasm flooding the phone line.

She seemed satisfied and I had her laughing before the conversation ended. We understood each other. We were both frustrated, and we were both getting very tired.

On January 12, Hospice came to the house and visited with Joy. It was agreed that given her situation, Kevin being able to come in and out during the day, and the fact that I could get to Teri's by mid-afternoon for a while before Teri got home and we could call an occasional "babysitter," 24 hour care would not be needed! Joy was very happy with that arrangement. Teri and I didn't feel quite as happy as she did because we felt better knowing someone was with her all the time, but we would just have to trust the Lord for this one!

New Year's came and now a new year is here. I spent the night with Sandy and Jim. God has given me another year and I praise Him.

Sandy's sister, Carolyn, and her daughter, Traci, and Traci's husband, Scott, came over to see Amanda and to take a drive in my car. I am going to sell my car to Scott. I would love that. It would sort of still be in the family. It is hard to sell it but I know that I must. I am getting a very fair price for it and Scott will take really good care of it. It makes me happy to sell it to someone who will enjoy it as much as I do. Traci and Scott will remember me every time they drive it! That thought will ease the pain of selling it.

My breathing is getting very difficult. I had a panic attack at the hospital and I thought I was going to die. I was so scared. I knew something was wrong. Teri and Sandy took me to see Dr. Beveridge on January 9. After looking at my latest heart test he told me that I would have to stop taking Herceptin, and the next two weeks I would just have to be in God's hands. Well, I've always been there! I will continue to trust the Lord. Teri and Sandy had a hard time with the news. I tried to stay strong for them. I didn't want to lose it. I know that God has the last decision. My life has always been in His hands and He knows when my time here on earth is finished.

Also, he told me that I would have to move in with Kevin and Teri for those two weeks and that he wants me to go into the Hospice program. I'm glad that Hospice will be coming to Teri's. I really don't want to go to a Hospice center. I know that I will have to start thinking about selling my condo. I guess when things start going downhill, they go down fast!

"Lord, I love you and I need you and I know you were with me in the beginning, and you will be with me in the end! I love you, Lord." I'm so tired. I can't write anymore.

Chapter 52

The Message Is Still Strong

When the Hospice nurse made her first visit to see Joy on January 12, she set her up with oxygen, which seemed to make Joy feel more comfortable, got all her medications ordered, and did an examination. Joy instantly liked her, gave her our book and, of course, witnessed to her. When she told Joy she would not need a "babysitter," that made Joy like her all the more! Hospice told Teri that they would send someone twice a week to monitor Joy and that we could get a private nurse to fill in the other times when that became necessary. Hospice also would arrange to have someone come in twice a week and help bathe and dress Joy if we desired that service. Teri and I discussed it and decided we would hold off on that until it was absolutely necessary, because we didn't want to take anything away from Joy!

Joy and I had made a commitment to speak at a breakfast for the Mount Vernon Church of the Nazarene on January 16. I wondered if Joy, due to her breathing difficulty, would be able to speak, but she insisted that she could. Zelda went with Joy, Teri and me. We took Joy into the church in her wheelchair and attached to her oxygen tank.

It didn't take long for me to relax and feel just fine about Joy. Her eyes fairly shone in that room and she looked perfectly peaceful even with the oxygen. When she was taken to the platform, she grabbed the microphone and started talking like she always had. For about fifteen minutes she gave her riveting testimony of God's grace in her life. And even when it was apparent to all that her breath was almost gone and she had to stop frequently to gather herself, she would not give up until she had told them what God

233

had laid on her heart. There were many tears on the cheeks of those who heard her that day. She had once again praised the Lord for another opportunity to serve Him, and had told that captive audience that if it had taken cancer to make her into the person God wanted her to be, then she would praise Him even for the cancer!

We left that place amazed at the strength God had given her, and I knew her testimony had once more changed lives.

As Teri and I spent the rest of the day painting her bedroom a very sunny yellow (her favorite color), I thanked God for the privilege that had been mine to care for this child of God, for I knew her reward would be great and my life had been made richer!

But we have this treasure in jars of clay to show that this all-surpassing power is from God and not from us. We are hard-pressed on every side, but not crushed; perplexed, but not in despair; persecuted, but not abandoned; struck down, but not destroyed. We always carry around in our body the death of Jesus so that the life of Jesus also may be revealed in our body.
— 2 Corinthians 4:7-10

I made it to the Nazarene Church breakfast for us to speak. I love speaking! I love to give my testimony. You could feel the spirit of the Lord in that room. I thank God for giving me the strength!

Sandy and Teri worked for days getting my bedroom ready. I have been sleeping in one of Teri's smaller bedrooms. The larger one has a bathroom in it. It is looking so nice. The girls are doing such a great job. They painted it yellow. They think it is too bright, but I love it! I would wheel in and out of the room and check it out. It was nice just to be able to watch them work for a change! Ha, Ha! That is what I told them. Best of all, they are doing it out of "love," and that is what makes it special for me. We all love each other and it shows!

I thank you all for making another memory for me to take with me. You all can have it as a memory some day, too.

Well, I'm tired now and I'm sure I will sleep well tonight because y'all wore me out!! Ha! I love you girls and thanks for making everything so nice for me. That goes for all of you guys, too, who did the heavy moving. I love you all!

Chapter 53

A Special Afternoon Sent By The Father

For those next two weeks, we just had to sit and watch. Some days Joy's breathing was good and some days it was not. Some days she looked good, and other days it looked like it might be her last.

The Hospice nurses came twice a week and monitored her breathing, heart and blood count. Joy opted to take as little pain medication as she possibly could. They left it entirely up to her. The nurse told us that most patients in her condition opted to have much more medication, but Joy was not "most patients." She wanted to have as clear a mind as possible.

Jim and I went over to Kevin and Teri's often to bring Joy to our house. It was difficult transporting the large oxygen tank with her; hooking it up and carrying her had become quite an ordeal. But we wanted her to feel as much a part of our family as we possibly could and so we managed. Kevin and Jim would struggle to get everything in the car when we picked her up at their house and they would struggle to get it all back into the house when we brought her home. They actually got pretty good at it.

We were able to take her to church the next Sunday, but before the end of the service, I had Adam go to the car and get the reserve tank of oxygen for her. She had become so dependent on it that she panicked whenever it got low! She enjoyed the service but it was obvious that it was too tiring on her, and she wouldn't be going too many more Sundays!

Joy had a doctor's appointment early on January 22. Teri and I went with her. Her heart sounded a little better to him, but he still didn't have any answers for us. He didn't know what else to do.

He looked puzzled and frustrated, but still amazed at Joy's smiling face!

Jim and I took Amanda, Julie and Rita to Old Towne Alexandria for lunch at Gadsby's Tavern later that day. It was last year almost the same time that Jim, Joy and I had taken Sherry there for lunch when she came to visit. We ate and laughed and even took in some sightseeing. It seemed like so much longer ago than one year. My memory of that lunch was bittersweet but then as I was brought back to the present, I looked over at my "girls" talking and laughing together and I praised God for our family. I knew that I could count on them to get me through those next few weeks — for I knew it was only weeks. Jim took Rita back to work and Julie, Mandy and I browsed in some quaint little shops, stopped by "Papa's" office for a visit, and then went home.

For a while that afternoon I felt normal. My heart sang. I laughed and giggled and it was as though I was in a completely different time and place, transported away from cancer, sorrow and death. It was almost euphoric.

Once home, reality set in again as I listened to the messages on our telephone answering machine. But as I held my tiny granddaughter in my arms and I watched her sleeping peacefully, I realized that God had given me that wonderful afternoon and it was His gift to me just as this baby was His gift — given as a healing balm for the hurts of the past few months, and the hurt that I knew was ahead for me. As I pulled Amanda closer to me and kissed her precious forehead, I praised God over again for His love and for His infinite grace and miraculous timing!

Chapter 54

The River Is Raging

Teri and I kept in contact several times a day. We constantly worried that something would happen when we were not there. We would soon need to hire a nurse for the daytime, but it had become apparent that we now had to have the help of an aide from Hospice three times a week. God sent a wonderful aide. Her name was Laverne and Joy loved her. We felt comfortable when she was there.

Although Joy didn't like to think of them as "babysitters," women from our church and other churches in the area came by on a regular basis just to drop in or to say, "Hello." She did appreciate that very much. Julie would bring Amanda, and Rita and Adam dropped by frequently. Andrew had a very difficult time. He visited, but it was painful for him — very painful. He felt so very helpless as we all did. But Andrew has always had a particularly painful time with letting go. His pain seems so much deeper than most of us suffer. Maybe it is because he has a hard time talking about it. He loved Joy like a sister. I prayed that God would comfort him.

Joy's medication was changed constantly because of her changing needs. We kept charts and carefully monitored her meds. She seemed more and more breathless to me, and her spirits were down for the first time. She was almost paranoid with the oxygen, for without it she felt as though she would suffocate. I knew that feeling very well, for last summer I had choked on a piece of steak and a friend had to perform the Heimlich maneuver on me to dislodge it. It was the most frightening thing I have ever gone through. I couldn't breathe and I was terrified! I knew she felt that same way much of the time. I prayed to God to take that feeling away from her — to let her breathe normally — not to let her suffocate!

I knew we were close to saying goodbye. I felt numb each time I saw her. I knew her time was close, and she knew it too. I longed to be able to close my eyes and when I awoke she would be in glory and we would have already gone through this process of "goodbye." My heart still ached from the long three-week-goodbye I had just gone through with my mother, not even one year ago! Now I had to face doing it again. But I knew that I would have the strength to face it when it came. I remembered Joy's words: "God doesn't build a bridge until we come to the river." I would have the strength when I got to the river!

Sherry and Debby called from Ohio on a regular basis to check on Joy's condition. They wanted to see her again, and Teri and I agreed that it had to be soon if they wanted to see her when she would remember who they were. Sometimes Joy's mind would get confused because of the cancer in her brain. Those times would scare us, but we knew it was all part of the process.

Sherry and Debby would arrive in Washington on February 11. It was the earliest they could come. Because of Scott's schedule, Debby had to wait until he could be there for their children before she could come. Joy seemed to understand that and she looked forward to their visit. I prayed that she would hold on long enough to see them.

I called my dear friend, Lou, in New York and Joy's friend, Brenda, as well as other friends far and near, and asked them to pray fervently for Joy that God would take her peacefully and without suffering. "Please, Lord. Please take her gently — very gently. Don't let her struggle for her breath, Lord. Please hear my prayer."

That river that we had to come to seemed now to be forming into a raging angry sea with huge waves crashing against the shore. "Is there a bridge high enough to cross that?" I asked God. Only He could take us across and in His arms He would have to carry us for neither she nor I could walk across — not this time!!

I went to church today, January 31, but it was hard. My breathing is hard. Kevin brought the big tank because I'm going to go over to Sandy and Jim's and watch the Superbowl with them.

Kevin struggles with all the stuff he has to do for me but he doesn't complain. You are loved, Kevin. Always be the same sweet guy and take care of Teri.

We had a nice day but I wish I could breathe without the oxygen. Sandy had to give me the drops a few times. They help me to breathe better.

Jim and Sandy took me home after the game. Jim struggled with that stupid oxygen tank, too. I love you, Jim. You are a gift to any woman! What a man and a father and husband you are! You put a lot of men to shame! You are my buddy!

No matter how difficult and painful my road, it is marked by the footprints of my savior. He has already been there. He is our forerunner. Each burden we have to carry was once placed on His shoulders. This comforts me to know that He has gone before me and He knows what I am going through this very minute. I must follow His way for He is my example. "Thank you, Lord, for always being there. Thank you for loving me so much."

Again, thanks, Teri and Kevin, for loving me. Ty, I hope you will remember me and that I loved you!

Chapter 55

Silver And Gold

I went to see Joy on the afternoon of February 1 to talk with her. We needed to have a real "buddy" talk. She agreed with me. It was a hard talk — very hard. She asked me if I thought she was dying now.

"Yes," I told her with tears in my eyes and a lump in my throat. "I think it is close now."

"So do I," she said softly in short gasps but without lifting her eyes to meet mine. "I know that God can still heal me if it is His will, but I think He wants to call me home soon."

"Are you tired?" I asked her as I held her hand and rubbed her back.

"Yes. I'm very tired," she replied, as she laid her head against my heart.

I could not keep the tears from flowing as I buried my head into her hair and pressed her close to me.

"Don't cry," she whispered. "It will be all right, I promise you. Promise me that you will be here for Teri. She will need someone to talk to and you are the best."

"I promise you that I will be here for her anytime she needs me."

"You know that if there is any way at all that I could come back and talk to you after the Lord takes me, that I would find it?"

"Oh, I am very sure that if there is any way at all, you would be the one to find it, Kiddo. How will I know it's you?" I said to lighten up our conversation. "Would I hear someone softly yelling 'football'?" That is what we would call out when we were in a place (like WalMart, for instance) where we had gotten separated from one another. It was a line from a funny movie we had seen together that had starred Goldie Hawn. We laughed and laughed at the scene we would make if she suddenly appeared from heaven yelling, "Football!" It was good to laugh — very good.

"All I know," she said as she hugged me tightly, "is that when I found you and Jim, I found gold and silver."

I laughed as I asked her through the cascading tears, "Yeah, but who is the gold?"

She smiled that still gorgeous smile and said, "You're the gold!"

Funny, but I felt a certain peace after we had that conversation, and I think that she did also. We needed to talk and we surely did need to laugh. It was painful, but the Lord had used it as a soothing balm for my soul.

Sandy came over this afternoon to sit for a while and talk. We talked about heaven. She rubbed my back and it felt so good. I rested my head on her lap. It felt good to have her hold me and make me feel safe. We talked and then we just sat together for a long time. I told her that sometimes I'm afraid to close my eyes and she prayed with me so that I will not be afraid. I don't know why I am afraid to do that — close my eyes. I'm not afraid of dying. My thinking is sometimes not so good now.

All of a sudden I'm getting very sleepy. I think I'll just close my eyes and lie down for a while.

Chapter 56

God Is Not Finished Yet

Joy began suffering panic attacks where she was convinced she could not breathe! These were scary episodes for Teri. She began spending the nights sleeping on the sofa just down the hall from Joy's room. She could look straight down the hall and see Joy. I worried about Teri because I knew she was having to get up at nights with Joy, and her sleep was constantly being interrupted.

Every time we called the Hospice nurse and she would come and check on Joy, she would assure us that things were normal considering Joy's condition, and that it was part of the process. They were constantly amazed that she had indeed lived as long as she had. Each time they came they would tell us that she only had a few days, or a week or so at the most. Those times would come and go and Joy was still here. God was in control and no one else. Joy continued to have good and bad days. Some days she would fight us and yell at us and give us a hard time when we tried to give her the medicine. Other times she was docile, cooperative and sweet. You never knew from day to day what she would be like. We knew that it was the cancer and though it hurt us to see her that way, we knew she wasn't herself.

One evening when Jim and I were visiting with Joy, she indicated that she needed to go to the bathroom and it was obvious to us that she had soiled her diaper for the umpteenth time that day! Teri looked exhausted but never complained about anything she was doing for Joy. She got up to take Joy to the bathroom, but I jumped up first and insisted on taking her. When we were there we tried to give Teri and Kevin a break as often as we could.

"Let me do the honors," I said to Teri as I winked and proceeded to put Joy into the wheelchair and take her down the hall and into the bathroom. After I cleaned her up and put fresh underwear on her, she sat back down to rest for a few minutes before we went back. It had become quite an ordeal just to get her into the bathroom and back to her chair again!

"Are you okay with this?" I said as I pointed to her head. "Up here. Are you okay?"

"Yes. I think I really am," she breathlessly answered. "Are you okay?"

"No!" I cried, with tears splashing down onto the sink. "I'm not okay. You know you are taking a piece of my heart with you."

"I know I am, but I'll only take a small piece. Okay?"

"Take care of it for me," I whispered in her ear as I told her I loved her.

"Don't start, Sandbox! I'll start crying and I don't have enough breath to cry," she said quietly as she gripped my hand hard and we began our long trip back to the living room.

I cried all the way home. Jim placed his arms around me and said, "She needs us now more than ever and you have to be strong. We have to be there for her." I felt my heart ripping apart again, and just when I thought it was beginning to heal.

I called and checked on our baby granddaughter when I got home. It was such a comfort for me to know that she was safe and sleeping. If I closed my eyes tightly I could feel the warmth of her body in my arms, and feel her heartbeat against mine. "Thank you for her, Lord." What did we ever do without her? How could a tiny baby become such a large part of your life in just a short amount of time, and provide healing that the mightiest of doctors could not? Only by the grace of God!!

Chapter 57

Tell Jesus I'm Coming Too

Joy was looking forward to Debby and Sherry's visit. It would be good for us to see them. Lou, our friend from New York, had wanted so much to come also, but things in her personal life prevented that from happening so she called frequently and cheered Joy up with her silly jokes and frivolous banter. Her phone calls made Joy laugh and were medicine just as surely as a visit.

Everyone that loved Joy wanted to do something. No one could "fix it," but everyone wanted to help, and everyone did just that — each one in his or her own way — everyone ministered love to Joy in a tremendous outpouring. She still had good and bad days, days when she seemed stronger than the day before, and days when she seemed to be very close to the end. However, she still loved having people visit, receiving gifts and cards, and calls. I know she felt their love.

Julie brought Mandy over to see Joy every couple of days. Joy would hold the baby until her arms were too tired to hold her any longer. Sometimes she just wanted Julie to lay the baby on her lap. I knew it made Joy very happy to have the time with Amanda. She told me over and over that she had prayed for God to allow her to live until she could see the baby. We had all prayed for that same thing.

Julie would fix lunch for Joy, and the two of them would watch a movie or just talk. Those times were very precious to Joy, and I was grateful to Julie for doing that.

Pastor Neil visited Joy regularly and prayed with her. Joy loved him and his family and she felt so much better when he visited. Our praise band came over one evening and we sang all of her favorite praise choruses. Pastor led in a short devotional and ministered communion to Joy and to us. It was a blessed evening and I was so happy that Joy seemed to have a pretty good command of the situation and was aware of what was happening. The presence of the Lord was certainly evident there. Joy was touched by the ministry.

Zelda spent time with Joy during that last month. Zelda had become like a grandmother to Joy and Joy loved her so much. Zelda just always seemed to know what to do and say. I always felt better after seeing Zel. She would sometimes be there to help Teri and me give Joy medication and do bedtime care. She often prayed with us. Each time Joy had company, especially those closest to her, they would leave her feeling as though they had seen her for the last time, because she seemed to be slipping away so rapidly.

I called Janet Parshall around the middle of the month to give her an update on Joy's condition and just to talk to her. We had both, Joy and I, felt as though Janet was our kindred spirit. We knew that she prayed for Joy and that she was concerned about us and what we were going through. She had requested that we keep her updated on Joy's condition. I called and left a message for Janet and she returned my call. How precious our conversation was as I poured out my heart to her and asked for her continued prayer.

"I will certainly be praying for the both of you and I know the Lord is guiding you through this, Sandy. You are a wonderful friend. God will bless you beyond measure for this. Tell Joy that I look forward to enjoying eternity with her and ask her to tell Jesus that I'm coming too!"

I know Janet is a very busy lady and for her to take the time to personally call me back and to give such encouragement, meant the world to me. I will never forget her for she is an angel that the Lord brought into our lives at just the right time. I told Joy of Janet's call. She smiled and said, "That Janet is so sweet. I love her. I'll tell Jesus what she said."

We all needed to tell Joy that — to ask her to tell Jesus that we are coming, too! It was a comfort for her to think about the "family" being all together once again. One day she told me that she would be waiting for me at the gate. I think she will — she will be right there waiting for me!

Julie came over with Brooke. She fixed lunch for us and we watched *Parent Trap.* I love that movie. It is so good!

I like you coming over, Julie. I love getting to know you better — just you and me. I got to know Rita so well when she stayed with me before their wedding and I loved that. Now I get to know you better, too. You are a good mom, and some day you and Andrew will stand back and look at your kids and see what a good job you have done with God's help. I will store the memories of the days you and I and Amanda are together! You will have them also, and they are good memories — happy ones! Thank you, Julie!

Chapter 58

The Sweet Fragrance Of Christ Filled The House

Joy's medication was changed again by Laura, the Hospice nurse; therefore, Joy was sleeping more. Teri and I felt like it was for the best because Joy had been very uncomfortable and very agitated most of the time before the change in medication. Now she seemed to be resting and breathing better and her mood was definitely improved.

It was clear that the cancer was affecting her brain more and more with every passing day. She forgot things regularly, her journals were becoming almost illegible and she could no longer talk on the telephone because her conversations were incoherent and jumbled much of the time. Still, at any given time, she could speak clearly and make perfect sense.

Debby and Sherry arrived on February 11. It was so great to see them and they were so glad that Joy recognized them. They spent almost all of their time with her. It was a welcome break for Teri and for me as well. They insisted on caring for Joy when they were with her, and they became quite proficient at it!

Teri and I discussed full time care for Joy. It was time to get a nurse to be with her during the day — all day. It had been working pretty well with Kevin popping in and out, Julie coming regularly, friends from church dropping by and my coming after work until Teri got home, but the time had come when we were afraid of leaving her alone at all! Joy was losing bladder and bowel control more often and her needs had become much greater. She wore diapers all the time, and was incapable of going to the bathroom alone. The women that had been coming and taking turns caring for Joy, were becoming alarmed now because of the changes occurring in Joy's condition. They still wanted to come, but felt incapable of providing the care that she needed. Some of them tearfully confided to me that they simply felt inadequate. I assured them that we understood perfectly and we were going to get full time care for Joy. They could still provide companionship, but without having to do her personal care and minister medication. It would be better all the way around! And indeed those blessed women continued to come and minister love and care to Joy up until the day God called her home!

Debby and Sherry didn't have a problem with providing Joy's personal care probably because they had known her so much longer than most of the women who had been sitting with her. They agreed to be with Joy full time for the time they were here. That gave us time to set something up with a nursing agency referred to us by Hospice. Those days they spent with Joy were invaluable to Teri and me. Joy enjoyed their being with her and she didn't mind the personal care they had to give her. With some people I know she felt uncomfortable as would we all. Cancer does strip you of your dignity! However, with Sherry and Debby it was different; they were like sisters.

The day came for Debby and Sherry to leave and Debby pulled me aside and said that she wanted to stay for another week. She and Sherry had discussed it. Sherry, although she wanted very much to be able to stay also, had to get back to her job. But Debby had already called Scott and they had agreed that if Debby could help us, she wanted to stay.

It was an answer to prayer, for by Debby staying with Joy for that next week, it gave Teri time to arrange for a nurse to come by the following Monday. Debby wanted to help and it couldn't have come at a better time!

With that settled, Debby, Jim and I drove Sherry to the airport and through a tearful goodbye she left and assured us that she was praying for us. She knew she would never see Joy again this side of heaven, but she had ministered love to Joy and that was something she could treasure forever!

Debby spent each day that week with Joy from early in the morning until Teri came home. It made Teri and me realize how much easier it was for us to work if we knew someone was with Joy all during the day. It also was good for Joy because she, too, realized that it was time to have full-time help.

Debby, Jim and I prepared dinner for Joy one evening and we insisted that Teri and Kevin go out for dinner! They needed a break and we agreed to keep Tyler with us. Reluctantly, they took us up on the offer, although when they returned we scolded them because they surely weren't gone very long!

After dinner, Debby and I readied Joy for bed. It had become an enormous chore. Joy's thought processes were not clear. She was becoming particularly beligerent with Teri and me at bedtime and during medication times. We constantly had to keep a sense of humor or we couldn't have made it.

While Debby straightened Joy's bed, I helped her with her shower. After I had her dressed for bed and changed her diaper, she reached out her arms to me and hugged me. She knew that she had been difficult but it was beyond her control. She fought back the tears because crying made her breathing so much more difficult.

"I love you!" she whispered.

"I love you, too." That was all that I could manage to say. Her dignity was going and that had been all she had left. It was the last thing that I know she wanted — to lose her dignity!

The next day, Joy lost her temper and took it out on Debby. "Welcome to the club," I told Debby. "It happens to Teri and to me on a regular basis. Just consider yourself in our elite club. We were beginning to think we were alone." Teri and I had joked after one particularly difficult night that if the Lord didn't take her home soon, we might be forced to send her to Him!! We truly had to keep each other sane! Debby, of course, took it in stride, and did not get upset at all. We laughed as she said she would pray extra hard for Teri and for me!

We were sorry to see Debby leave at the end of that week but we felt so blessed to have had her for so long. She cried when we took her to the airport, but I know she wouldn't have missed that week for the world. She would never know how much she had done for all of us. I agreed to keep her informed on a regular basis and, of course, we knew we were assured of her prayers. People all over the country were indeed praying for us and we could feel those prayers as never before.

God's word tells us in 2 Corinthians 2:15, *"As far as God is concerned there is a sweet, wholesome fragrance in our lives. It is the fragrance of Christ within us, an aroma to both the saved and the unsaved all around us"* (Living Bible). All those who ministered to Joy, filled that house during those long weeks with the sweet fragrance of Christ, each one giving of his or her God-given gifts to a child of God weakened in the battle. You know who you are. I haven't room to mention all of your names and even if I tried, I would surely miss someone. You will never know just how much your love was felt and cherished by not only Joy, but by Teri and her family and me and my family. God will richly reward you for your service to Him.

Chapter 59

Job's "Friends"

Try as we would, we could not please everyone. It amazed me that people who otherwise knew nothing about medicine could suddenly become experts in the field as they questioned us about our care for Joy: the medicine dosages were wrong, shouldn't she be in the Hospice facility, why weren't we making her eat, why was she confused (it must be the medicine!) — and on and on.

Hospice assured Teri and me that this was a normal reaction of people who didn't have a clue! Joy was being carefully monitored by Hospice and they constantly assured us that we were doing everything right. The criticism was particularly difficult on Teri because she had to take most of the calls and, of course, because Joy lived at her home, she had the personal encounters with these "well-meaning friends." With the lack of sleep that Teri was getting at night, her nerves were really quite frazzled and to receive those calls (one at 11:30 p.m.), was most difficult on her. She called me the day after the late night call, crying and questioning herself. We talked for a long while and reasoned that these people, as Hospice had said, truly did not have a clue and we had to let it go and concentrate on Joy and just follow the Hospice instructions as we continued in constant prayer for wisdom. We laughed at their suggestions, for if we had listened to some of them we would have surely overdosed Joy many times over or, worse, killed her!

Thankfully, those "friends of Job" were few and the vast majority of our true friends were most supportive and so very helpful, kind and compassionate.

I have come to realize through the experience with the deaths of my mother and Joy, that unless you have walked in someone else's shoes, you really should not condemn or judge the caregiver. Some of the most difficult decisions of my life were made during the final days of my mother and Joy. Decisions such as: life support; surgery or not; feeding tubes; food and water in general, given or not to the dying patient; medications; nursing home or not; Hospice facility or home; were only a few of the heartbreaking decisions that had to be made. They were not easy decisions and with each one, I cried a thousand times and my heart broke into a thousand pieces. I didn't need condemnation. I needed support, prayer, love and understanding.

I grew during these past few years. I will never be the same, and I know that I have a far better understanding of death and dying than I once did. I hope that through my experience, I can help someone else who may some day be faced with having to make one or more of those same heartbreaking decisions for I, too, perhaps once judged as did Job's friends.

Job replied to the Lord in Job 42:1-3: *"I know that you can do all things; no plan of yours is thwarted. You asked, 'Who is this that obscures my counsel without knowledge?' Surely I spoke of things I did not understand, things too wonderful for me to know."*

The caregivers are often much more fragile than their patients. They should wear a sign that reads "Fragile — Handle With Care." May each of you who read the pages of this book remember and ask the Lord to help you to minister not only to the afflicted but to their caregivers as well! As is written in Psalm 147:3, you will surely help Him to *"heal the brokenhearted and bind up their wounds."*

Chapter 60

Close To Home

The tumors on Joy's spine were very visible the more weight she lost. Laura, the Hospice nurse, told us that we should offer food to Joy or encourage her to eat only if she wanted to eat, not to force her or worry if she didn't eat. Actually, she explained, the cancer was now using any food in Joy's body to feed itself! It was a frightening thought — the cancer actually eating even the nutrients that we were trying to give Joy for survival. For the first time I pictured the cancer as a living organism, vile and deceptive, and slowly killing its victim by even stealing her food! And yet, the one thing it can never steal is the soul and spirit of that victim unless the victim chooses to allow that, and Joy had not and would not!

Joy was becoming more and more confused but seemingly not in a lot of pain for which we were grateful. Teri and I were careful when we moved her because that seemed to be her greatest fear — the fear that we would drop her. Also the pressure against her spine, if we weren't careful, caused her back to hurt. The worst thing were times when she would not recognize us and then become frightened. She would fight us. Once she spit at me and hit Teri. Teri and I understood and loved her the more because we knew it wasn't her, and we knew it would have killed her to have known what she had done!

At other times, Joy would grab us, and tell us not to leave her, and how much she loved us. One evening she looked at me and said, "You've signed on with a new man!" The fear in her eyes, and the sound of her voice, made her sit straight up in bed.

"No, I haven't," I told her in an indignant voice!

"Yes, you have, and I can't believe you did that!"

Jim walked in just then and stood at her bedside holding her hand.

"See there! Jim is right here. I didn't take up with another man. I've given him too many years of my life to change now," I replied, trying to lighten the situation.

She laid back in the bed and smiled. She then told me it was time to "open the store." I told her that we would open the store, but she needed to sleep first.

These types of conversations were becoming more the norm. We had learned just to keep her as calm as we possibly could and get her to sleep. Most of the time she reverted to reality when she would awaken. Usually she never remembered anything about those crazy times and we never found it necessary to ask her about them for it would only have made her more convinced that she was losing her mind.

Our kids (even Andrew) kept making visits, but each visit during those last two weeks of her life was agony for them. I know that the recent death of my mother weighed heavily on their minds as they watched Joy literally fading away before their eyes. Sometimes she recognized them, but at other times she didn't or she slept much of the time they were with her. Friends popped in often to inquire as to what they could do, bring food, or just to let us know they were with us. You could hear hearts breaking with every visit and phone call.

With each goodbye to Teri, I wondered if the next time I heard her voice she would be telling me that Joy had gone home. I always hated to leave in the evenings because I didn't want Teri to be alone when Joy was taken. I knew full well that she would not be alone for the Lord was with her and there were angels surrounding Joy prepared to take her home when the Lord called.

"... I will never leave you or forsake you" (Hebrews 13:4) was never impressed upon me as surely as it was during those dark trips home after leaving Teri's house in the evenings. As I shed those bitter tears and called out to the Lord, I felt His mighty presence.

Chapter 61

Forever Friends

The first day of March found Julie and Amanda sick with very bad colds. Amanda had to have the nebulizer every four hours. The whole family was taking turns helping Julie and Andrew with the baby. It was hard for Julie to do it all when she herself was so sick. Rita was just recovering from a cold also. I was trying to care for all of them with my homemade chicken soup and TLC, while still helping Teri with Joy. Actually with the family needing me, I was able to keep my mind occupied — not as much time to dwell on the inevitable!

One evening Jim, Adam and I went to see Joy, and as I helped Teri get her ready for bed Joy looked up into my face and I knew she recognized me as she touched my cheek and said, "You are my best friend, you know?"

"Yes, I know that. We are best friends."

"Forever?" she said in a sleepy voice.

"Forever!"

"Then please take me home with you. I want to go home."

She gripped my hand hard and fell asleep. I prayed that the Lord would take her home. She was ready to go home and I was ready too. I was ready to let her go!

Oh a friend's a friend forever when the
Lord's the Lord of them.
And a friend will not say "never" 'cause the
Welcome will not end.
Oh, it's hard to let you go, but in the
Father's hands we know, that a lifetime's
Not too long to live as friends.

Michael W. Smith

Chapter 62

In His Own Time

Joy could not sleep! She just could not! Teri was up and down every night with her. The restlessness and lack of sleep were causing her to have pain. The Hospice nurse ordered Nembutal for Joy. It was to be given rectally every twelve hours. It was the only thing they thought would work, and Laura told us we had to do everything we could to get her to sleep.

The worst case scenario of the side effects of the Nembutal would be that it would hasten her death. She could die within two hours of the first dose! Dr. Beveridge was called and it was decided that it was absolutely the best for Joy. Teri and I cried as we had the medicine ordered. I promised Teri that we would do it together.

I arrived at Teri's at 3:00 the afternoon of March 2. "How are you today?" I said to Joy as I gave her a kiss and a hug.

"Okay for a country girl," she replied with almost a twinkle in her very tired eyes.

Joy slept until 4:30. Teri and I talked and waited for the medicine to arrive. It arrived at 5:00.

"Today is my day to die!" Joy said to our surprise as we went into her room to change her diaper. "Please change me. I don't want to die in wet clothes."

It was all we could do not to burst into tears as we helped her to the bedside commode. She pulled me down to her and told me she could see chariots. She told me that she loved me and that I was still her best friend. She pulled Teri down also and told her to hold onto the cross. "Carry the cross, Teri, and always remember that I loved you like a sister."

I honestly believed the Lord was going to take her right then and there. She wanted us to stay with her as she cried softly, "Please lie down with me — both of you."

We got her back into her bed, and she insisted that Teri get on one side of her and I get on the other side. We crowded into that small bed and as she held us close I began to talk to her about heaven. She agreed that it would be full of flowers, especially roses, like the ones in our garden, and that the sky would be bright blue. I asked her to save me a place in the choir and she said that she would.

"Do you see Him yet, Joy?" I asked her through tears.

"Not just yet, but I know He is beautiful."

I prayed God would please take her just then, but it was not to be. She drifted off to sleep and her breathing, which had been very labored, seemed to be more even.

Zelda arrived at 7:00 as did Jim. Zelda wanted to be with us when we administered the Nembutal to Joy. She thought we might need her, and we did.

"I just can't do it, Sandy," Teri cried before we entered Joy's room. "I just can't. I know we have to and I want to, but I can't." Teri sobbed as she held onto me, and her eyes begged the question that she could not ask.

The blood ran cold in my veins as I realized that it was up to me! I would have to give her the medicine that could, in fact, take her life within two hours! I looked at my friend lying there, and I realized that she really wasn't there. I believe the Lord had already taken a part of her unto himself. I would have been less than a friend if I had not done everything I could in order to make her last days, or perhaps hours, as comfortable as possible. I was tired of seeing her restless, in distress and confused. She would not have chosen that way to end her life. And so after Zelda prayed with us, I administered the Nembutal to Joy, removed my gloves, and sat down on the bathroom floor and cried.

Zelda rubbed Joy's back and spoke to her in soothing tones. Teri came to me and we just sat there in the floor and cried on each other's shoulders.

"You can't break down, Sandy. You have to stay strong for me. I need you so much." Teri sounded like a frightened child, as I assured her once again that we would get through this together. We waited two and then three hours and Joy slept — still restless, still seemingly discontent. Nothing had changed — nothing at all. Sound sleep still evaded her. I knew God had a purpose for this delay in Joy's homegoing even though it was not clear. Jim and I stayed until Joy finally settled down sometime after 10:30.

I felt totally exhausted after the ordeal as were Teri and Zelda. But it was in God's hands and we would only follow His lead. I prayed once again for strength for us all!

Chapter 63

The Angels Are Ready

On March 3, Teri and I began making funeral arrangements for Joy when the Hospice nurses told us they were certain that Joy could live only a week at the most. Joy had already made it abundantly clear what she wanted. She had filled out a booklet that she had received at the cemetery over a year ago, and she had recorded all of her wishes in writing. In fact, we had to laugh as we read some of her entries. For instance, one question that was asked regarding funeral plans was "Do you want a visitation?" Joy wrote a note beside that question: "What is this? I'm dead!" You had to know Joy to appreciate her sense of humor!

She also wanted as little money as possible spent on a funeral. We had all (including my mother) purchased burial sites at a nearby cemetery, Mount Comfort. We chose to be buried in the mausoleum because the cost was lower. We also selected the top tier in the mausoleum because it was the least expensive. We always referred to them as being located in the "sky suite"! We said that way our bodies would be closer to heaven when the rapture occurred. When Joy answered a question in the booklet concerning the cemetery site she had chosen, she listed the location of the site as being in the "sky SWEAT." Teri and I laughed as we read that. Joy's spelling was atrocious. She was forever calling me at work and asking me how to spell certain words. It had become a joke. She called me "Miss English"! Even in her death, she was giving us another glimpse of her spunk and spirit. We would miss that — sorely miss that!

We made all the pre-arrangements that we could. Joy wanted a memorial service that was filled with praise music and hope.

She wanted Jerry, one of our praise band members, and Adam as well as my sister, Carolyn, to sing and she even chose the songs they were to sing. She wanted our praise band to sing all her favorite praise choruses: "Sandy, you know the ones I love," she wrote in her notes. She wanted a sermon that would present the gospel in case people were there who didn't know the Lord. Above all, she didn't want a sad service. She made me promise on the day of her mother's funeral that I wouldn't let her service be sad, and that was the way Teri and I planned it — her way!

Joy continued to have good and bad days and nights. Some days she would sleep the entire day. Other days, she seemed restless and confused.

Rita was very sick and she spent most of the first week of March with us because Adam had to go to California for his job and Andrew had accompanied him. It was good for them to be away. There was nothing they could do, and they needed to be together. Julie and Amanda spent most of the week with us also. It was good for us to be together, also. Family had never meant so much as it had during the homegoing of my mother, and now awaiting Joy's call home, it was again very special!

On March 8, Joy told the Hospice nurse that she was "ready to finish the race." Her medication was increased and she seemed to be resting easier. It had been Joy's decision from the beginning to keep her medication at a minimum so that she wasn't "crazy," as she put it. Hospice honored her request, and meds were increased only when it was evident to Hospice that she had to have it increased or when Joy's pain became too much for the lower dosages to handle. She, in fact, had handled her own treatment from 1991 almost up until the end! She and Dr. Beveridge had an agreement, as did she and Hospice. They respected her opinions and her decisions. It had been apparent for the past few weeks that she was now way beyond making those decisions. Teri and I had to do that for her, and any way we chose seemed bitter!

Joy told Kevin one evening near the end: "I need to go, Kevin. Tyler needs me to go. He is afraid. I don't want him to see me like this. I need to go." Kevin assured Joy that he would take care of

Teri and Tyler, and that she could be sure of that. She seemed to understand that and she actually appeared to rest better that evening.

The end was near! I could almost hear the Lord calling her home. In His time He would call her unto Himself!

Chapter 64

The Race Is Finished

During the week of March 7, Teri brought work home every night as she had been doing ever since Joy had gotten worse. She faced a deadline, and she was trying to meet it. It had been hard on Teri over these past two months with trying to work a demanding full time job while also caring for Joy, especially when Joy hadn't been sleeping through the night for some time. At times I didn't know how she was managing. At least I could sleep through the night! I helped that week as much as I could, going over to stay with Joy every day after work from the time the nurse left at 3:00 until the time Teri came home from work, then returning after dinner to help get Joy ready for bed.

I had my devotions Thursday morning, March 11, and after talking to Julie she told me she had read the exact same devotional. It dealt with the miraculous burning bush Moses encountered on one seemingly ordinary day. That day God spoke to Moses and Moses stood on holy ground. Moses had taken the time to turn aside. I had been so busy with "things" that I hadn't taken time to turn aside and enjoy a personal visit with my Lord. The Lord wants us to draw closer to His heart of love and care. First Peter 1:8 says: *"Though you have not seen Him, you love Him; and even though you do not see Him now, you believe in him and are filled with an inexpressible and glorious joy."* In quietness we need to listen to Him — listen for His comfort or His healing balm.

Julie and I had been talking just a few days earlier about the need for our daily devotions, and she had confided to me that she didn't always take the time to have them every morning. I told her that I believe that is my greatest weakness. I seem to find a

271

multitude of reasons why I don't have time, and then when I start taking the time, I realize that my day goes so much better, and without fail, of course, God's word contains exactly what I need for the day! We purposed to keep each other accountable to do that!

I so needed those words that God gave me that Friday morning. God used them to prepare me for the next two days.

My devotion for March 12 was based on Romans 8:31: *"... If God is for us, who can be against us?"* We need to recognize that He is always for us — when we hurt, when we fail, when we are misunderstood, when our heart is breaking. When life is going smoothly, it is easy to say we love Him. The test is how much we love Him when the going is rough — when life is falling apart.

Joy slept for almost all of Friday and Saturday, March 12 and 13. Teri worked quietly at home on her computer, just down the hall from Joy's room. I called several times to check on Teri but she really didn't need me because Joy was sleeping most all of the time!

On March 13, I visited with Teri for a bit in the evening but Joy slept on. The last two days had been her most fitful sleep in at least two months. She hardly wakened even when we gave her a sponge bath or changed her diaper and clothing. Teri went in after Jim and I had gone for the evening to kiss Joy and tell her goodnight. Five-year-old Tyler decided that he wanted to help Teri. He was generally kind of reluctant to go into Joy's room, because Joy, who was always his playmate, couldn't play anymore, and it was a little scary to him seeing her sick. But this evening he chose to help his mommy. Teri had Joy's praise music on the stereo and Tyler was jumping around singing and clapping his hands. "I love you, Joy!" he was yelling loudly. "I love you."

Joy, who had not opened her eyes for two days, suddenly opened them and tried to speak. Most definitely she tried to tell him that she loved him, too. Teri and Tyler then kissed her goodnight and told her once again that they loved her. The next morning, March 14, 1999, Joy awoke at 7:00 in heaven. What better way to leave this world than to hear the words, "I love you," spoken over praise music!

The scripture in our devotional for that morning was miraculous and thrilling for all of us who knew and loved Joy. Timothy 4:6-8:

For I am already being poured out like a drink offering, and the time has come for my departure. **I have finished the race, I have kept the faith.** *Now there is in store for me the crown of righteousness, which the Lord, the righteous Judge, will award to me on that day — and not only to me, but also to all who have longed for his appearing.*

You do not choose your own cross. Your cross is prepared and appointed by divine love. Accept it cheerfully. Take up your cross as a follower of Jesus Christ. Don't run away in fear.

Jesus was a cross-bearer, and we could not have a better guide. The cross is not made of feathers or covered with velvet. It is heavy and cuts into disobedient shoulders. It is a heavy wooden cross but we can carry it because the Man of Sorrows knows its weight. Take up your cross and by the power of the Spirit of God you will soon be in love with it.

I read the above paragraphs somewhere but I don't remember where I found it. I love it! Everyone has a cross to bear and we don't all bear the same cross. My cross is cancer. I didn't always love my cross but I learned to love it because the Father uses it to make me into the person He wants me to be. If it took cancer to do that, then I praise Him for my cross.

You may be going through a dark room but remember, Jesus went through it before you. You may be facing a difficult fight but Jesus has faced the same enemy. Christ has carried the burden and His blood stained footsteps can be seen on the Road we are traveling.

Blessed is any storm that drives us closer to our Savior's Love. And blessed are the wounds that make us seek the Great and Beloved Physician.

If you can't bear the cross, you will never wear the crown!

***

These were Joy's favorite thoughts and the last notes written in her notebook! I don't know where she found the first few paragraphs but they meant so much to her. She was convinced that you could truly find joy in the Christian life by learning to love your cross. She lived each day just that way and she surely experienced abundant joy even in the midst of her cancer!

I introduced Joy to the Lord when she was fourteen years old and I taught her how to live, but through her life she taught me, and countless others, how to die! For that, I will be forever grateful. I'll meet her at the gate when I exchange, as Joy did, my cross for a crown!

If you are interested in having Sandy speak to your church, your women's organization or retreat, please contact her through Dr. Louise Neilsen by calling toll free at 1-877-478-7828 at Coping With Crisis Through Christ.

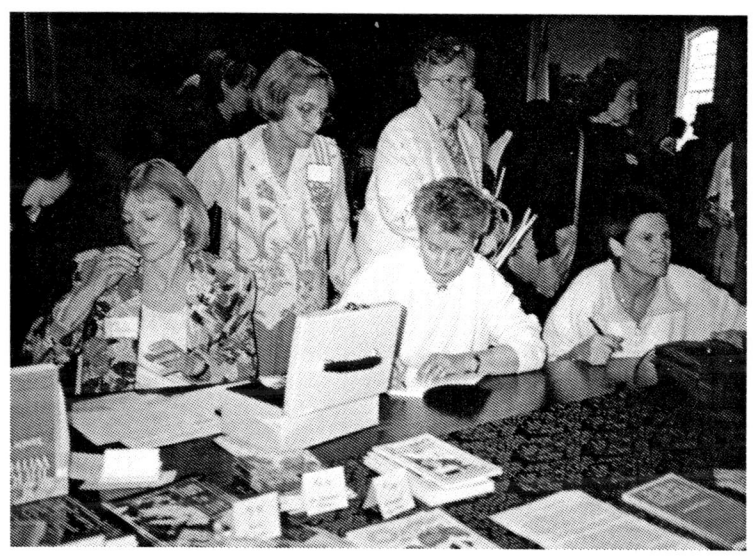

A book signing — Debby, Sandy, Joy — 1997

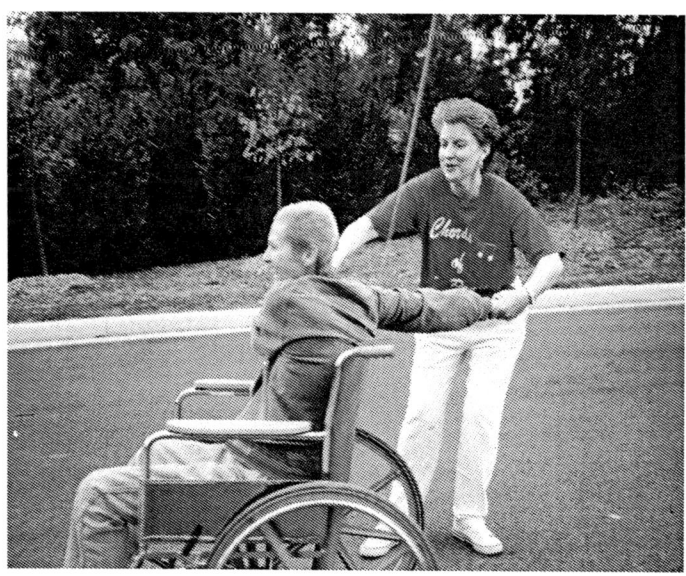

Do-si-do at the Block Party at Faith EPC — October 1998.

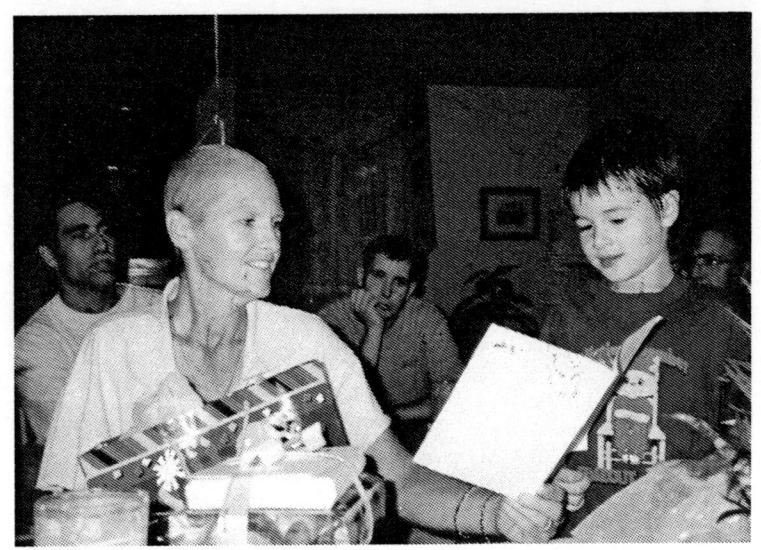

"Happy birthday, Joy." Joy and Tyler — July 1998.

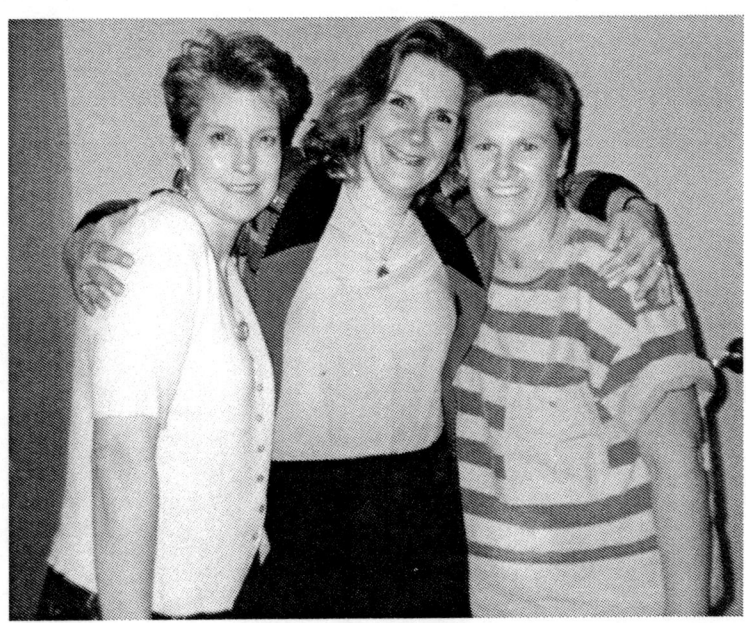

We are on "Janet Parshall's America." Sandy, Janet Parshall, Joy —
May 1997.

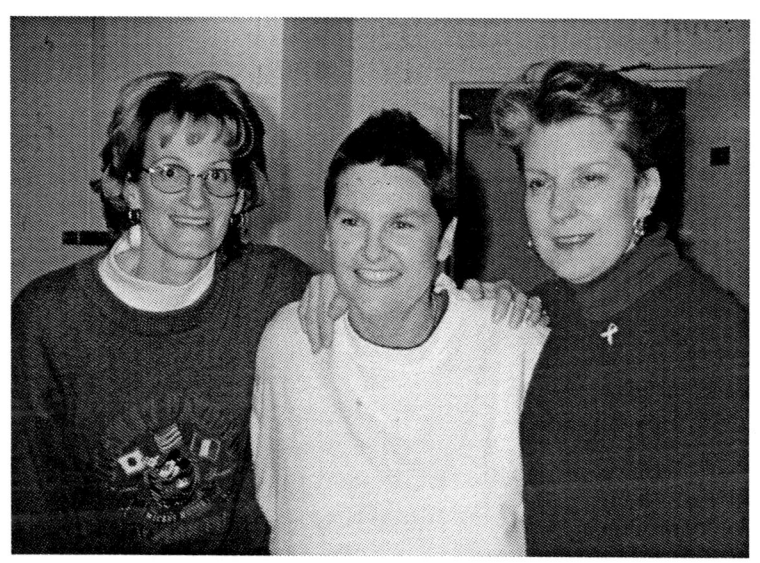

Teri, Joy, Sandy — February 1998

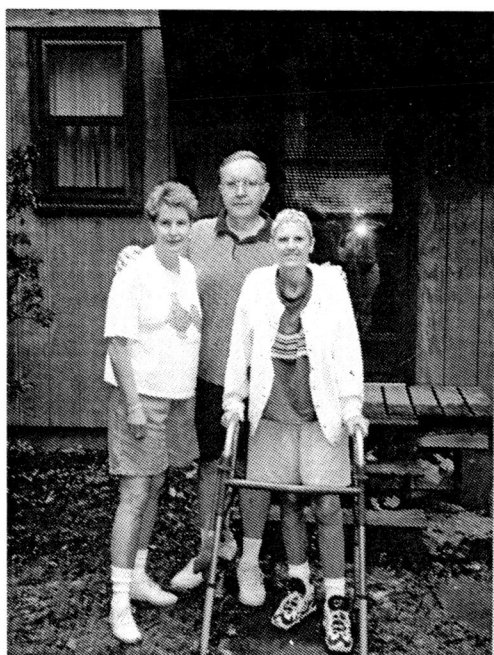

In LuRay, VA, Jim, Joy, and Sandy — August 1998.

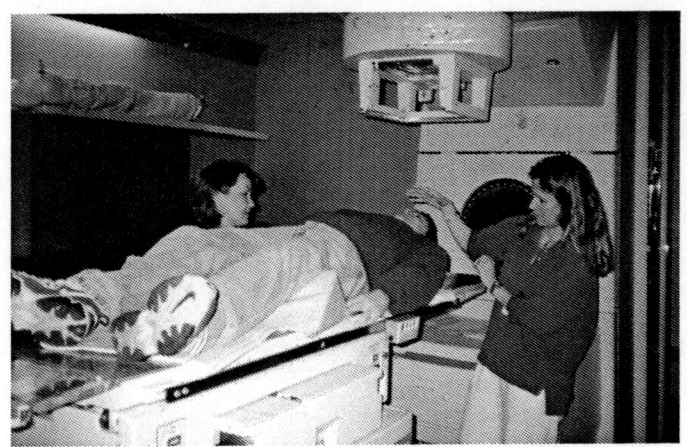

Joy's brain scan — "See what a small brain she has, Sherry." — February, 1998

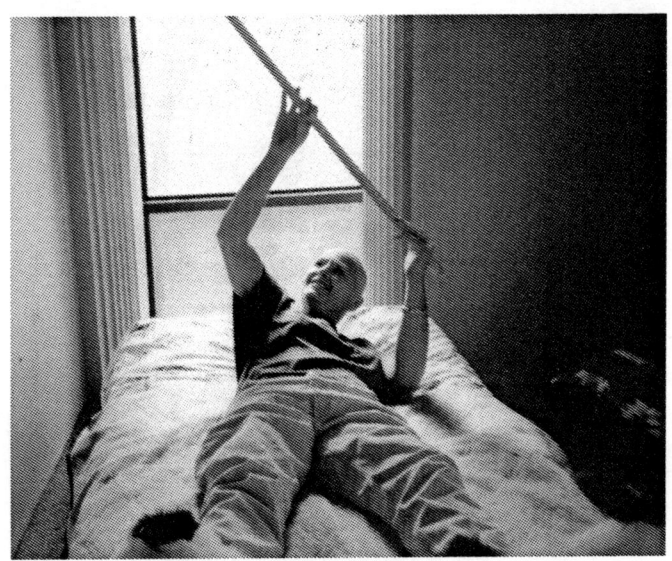

"Keep on painting," at the beach — June 1998.

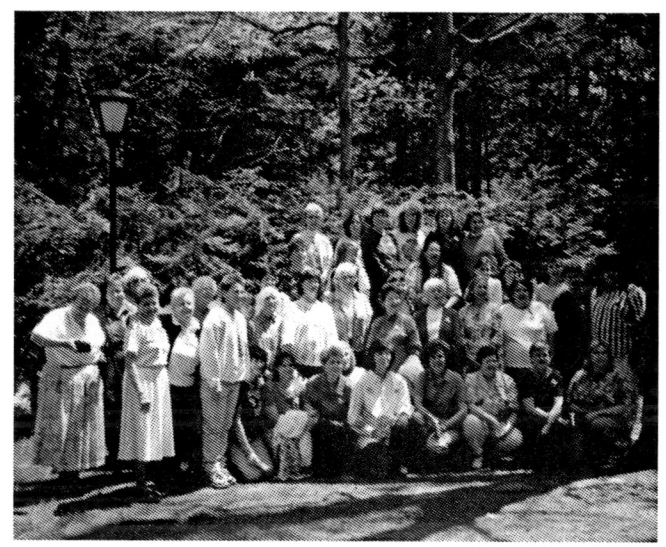

Our first "Speaking" Retreat — Evangelical Presbyterian Church — May 1997.

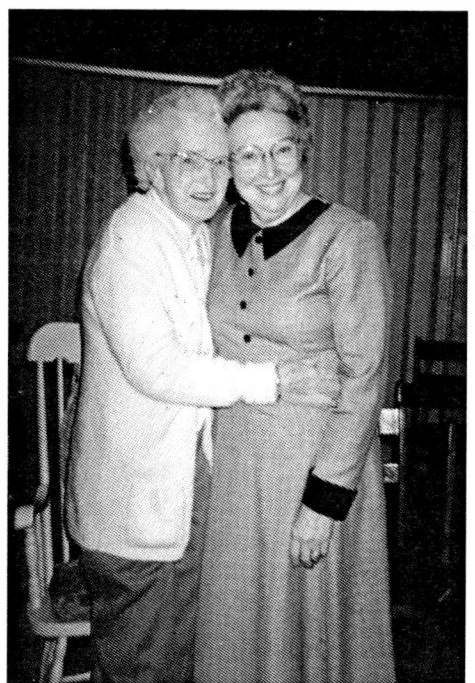

"Nina" and Patty Upshaw — Mom comes to a book-signing.

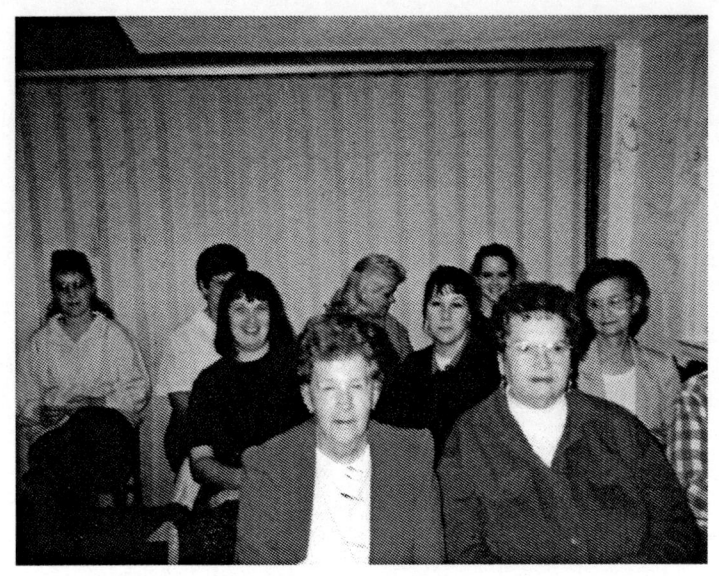

Our second favorite church — Rose Hill Baptist — February 1997. Our first book-signing.

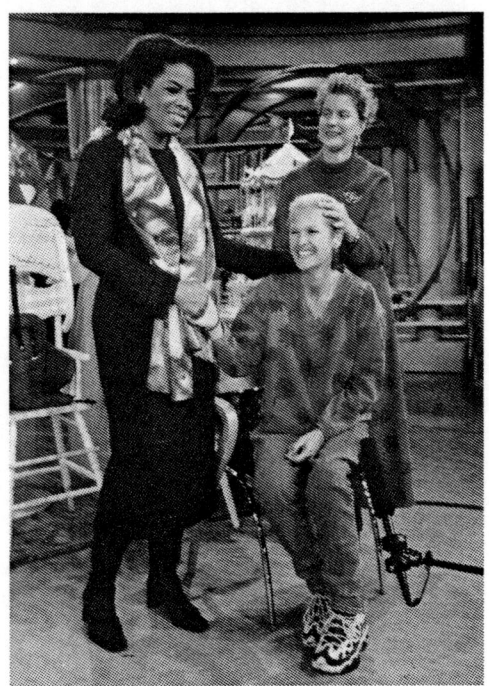

We meet Oprah — November 1998.
© 1998 Harpo Productions, Inc. All rights reserved.

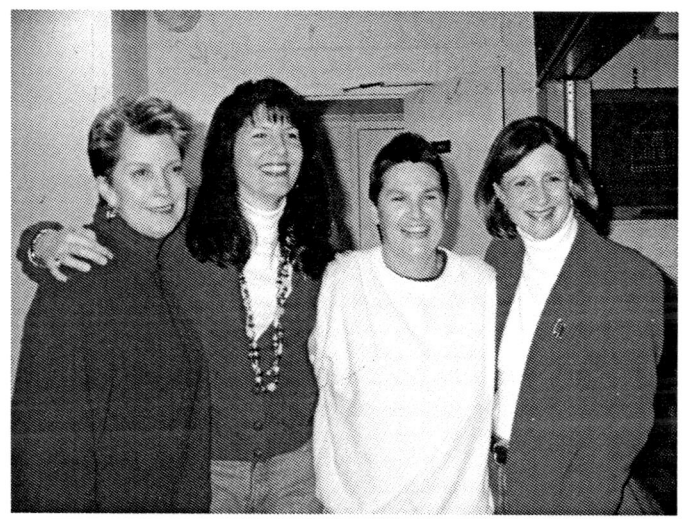

Sandy, Sherry, Joy, Debby. We speak at Rose Hill Baptist again —February 1998.

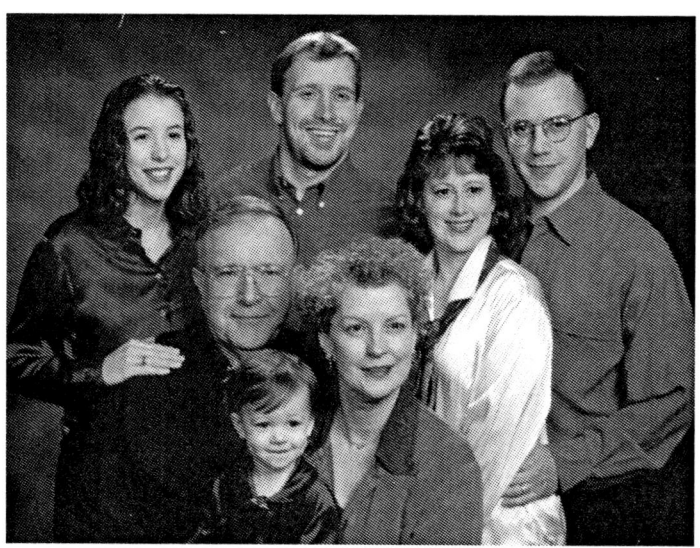

The Rice's — December 2000 — Amanda, Papa, Gigi, Rita, Adam, Julie, Andrew.

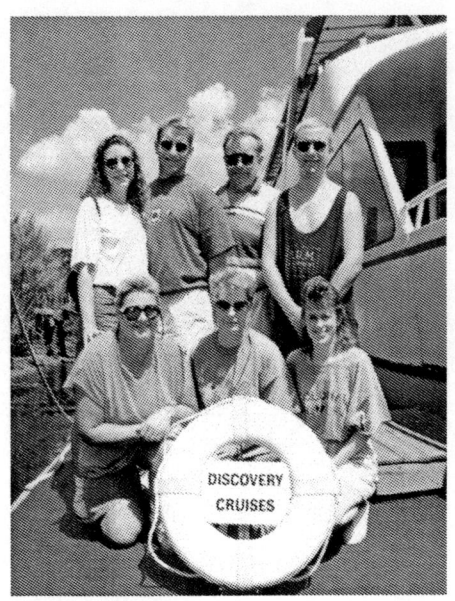

"We sail together." —June 1996

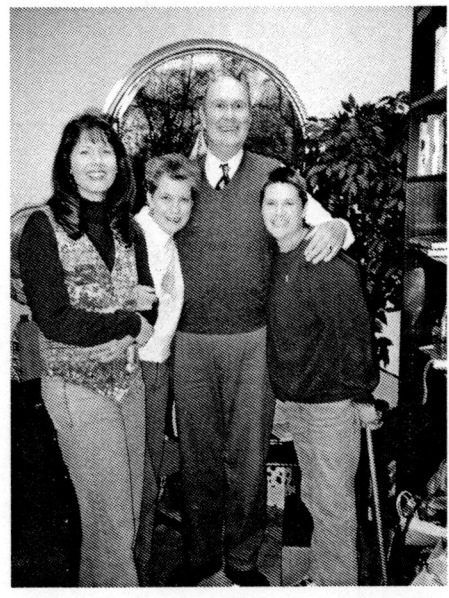

Sherry Neuenschwander, Sandy, Willard Scott, Joy

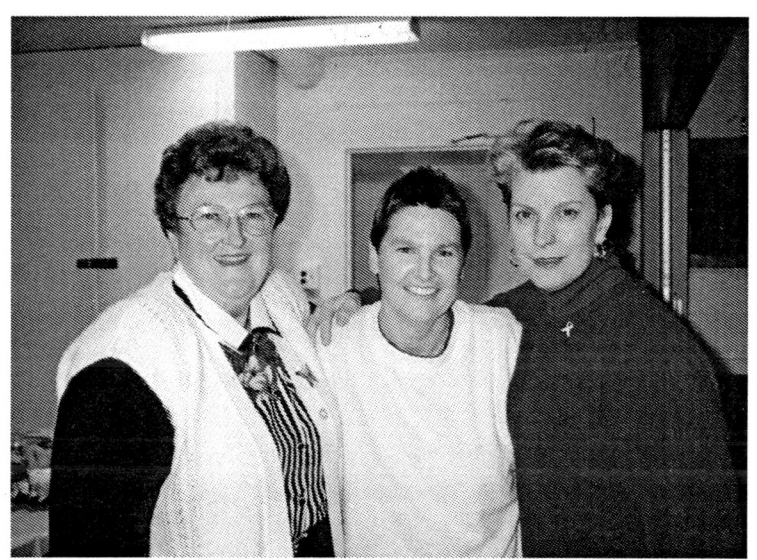

Zelda, Joy, Sandy — February 1998.

Photos on back cover: top — Joy and Amanda Brooke
bottom — Joy and Sandy